Don Mordasini, MA, MFT

Wild Child
How You Can Help Your Child with Attention Deficit Disorder (ADD) and Other Behavioral Disorders

D1472645

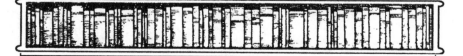

The Haworth Press
New York • London • Oxford

Wild Child

*How You Can Help Your Child
with Attention Deficit Disorder (ADD)
and Other Behavioral Disorders*

Wild Child

How You Can Help Your Child with Attention Deficit Disorder (ADD) and Other Behavioral Disorders

Don Mordasini, MA, MFT

The Haworth Press
New York • London • Oxford

The Haworth Press, Inc., 10 Alice Street, Binghamton, NY 13904-1580

This book should not be used as a substitute in place of psychotherapy for the treatment of attention deficit hyperactivity disorder or other mental disorders. The reader should consult a physician for matters relating to symptoms that may require medical attention. The case studies and vignettes presented in this book are based on actual clinical cases. However, all names, genders, and ages have been changed to protect the privacy of those individuals.

Cover design by Jennifer M. Gaska.

Library of Congress Cataloging-in-Publication Data

Mordasini, Don.
    Wild child : how you can help your child with attention deficit disorder (ADD) and other behavioral disorders / Don Mordasini.
        p. cm.
    Includes index.
    ISBN 0-7890-1101-8 (alk. paper) — ISBN 0-7890-1102-6 (pbk. : alk. paper)
    1. Attention-deficit hyperactivity disorder—Popular works. 2. Behavior disorders in children—Popular works. 3. Conduct disorders in adolescence—Popular works. 4. Child rearing. I. Title.

RJ506.H9 .M662 2000
618.92'8589—dc21

                                                                                    00-040735

to

My mother, Dorothy Mordasini, who was afraid to answer the door when the kids yelled, "Donny's hurt again." She loved me in my slowness, when I was put back a grade in school, when I was in trouble for gambling in the boy's john in the sixth grade, and later when I stayed out all night. Her stern words, "Wear your galoshes," "Put a scarf around your neck," I carry in my heart today. I give her thanks for teaching me unconditional acceptance.

to

My daughter Monika, who softened me with her glorious affection and adoration. She made love sooo *easy*.

to

My daughter Beate, who I virtually forced to ski avalanche mountains in the Alps, ever at her dad's side, even though she chewed me out when we got home. Her grace and beauty made love sooo *easy*.

to

My daughter Manuela, who made love so goddamn difficult with her own ADD. I give her thanks for *stretching* me to look beyond behavior to find the pearls inside.

to

Shri Ananda Ma, the universal embodiment of love, who taught me to find the divine incarnated throughout the creation.

My special appreciation to God as feminine, who wore all those faces for me and somehow maneuvered through my masculine rigidity so that I might pass on some of the gifts I received.

ABOUT THE AUTHOR

In 1983, **Don Mordasini, MA, MFT,** was a successful and rising star in the professional world—a vice president with Dean Witter Reynolds—and climbing the corporate ladder. In that year he experienced an emotional breakdown that culminated not only in a twenty-year marriage unraveling, but also in his giving up his professional career. He spent the next several years searching for who he was, trying to put the pieces together. It was at that time that he learned he had ADD.

Today, Don is a noted ADD psychotherapist, an area to which he brings a unique perspective, not only as an ADDer himself, but also as the father of an ADD daughter. As a partner in the highly respected Los Gatos Therapy Center, which is on the leading edge of ADD work, Don treats children, adolescents, and adults for ADD and its typical attendant disorders, anxiety and depression.

Don holds a bachelor's degree from the University of California at Berkeley. He is also a graduate of the Naval Officer Candidate School, and the Goethe Institute in Munich, Germany. In addition, he holds a master's degree from the Professional School of Psychology in San Francisco.

CONTENTS

Foreword

The entire subject of attention deficit hyperactivity disorder (ADHD) presents itself daily in newspapers, on television, on talk radio, and on the Internet. Exciting and significant advances are being made in the understanding of ADHD. Therapists, physicians, teachers, and even politicians are expressing many concerns about underdiagnosing or overdiagnosing, undertreatment or overtreatment. Health insurance company policies, HMOs in particular, and dwindling monies for mental health treatment reimbursement have led to shorter and less costly evaluations and treatments for children with ADHD. This often results in giving children medication only, or in not treating them at all. This shortsighted and inadequate approach does a tremendous disservice to these needy children and to their parents who often end up with merely a pill as their only means of professional help. The pill or no pills at all approach ignores the need to change ADHD children's long-standing maladaptive behavioral patterns developed in a desperate attempt to cope with their chaotic ADHD world. Also lost is the opportunity to help the parents of these children view ADHD with more understanding and change their parenting approaches.

In this current, sometimes confusing ADHD arena, it is timely and refreshing to be redirected, reorganized, and better grounded by Don Mordasini's new book, *Wild Child.* It is a remarkable, no-nonsense, practical, helpful guide for children and adolescents with ADHD, for their parents, and for therapists in the field. The book emphasizes what constitutes the condition and how misdiagnosis or undertreatment with medication alone can harm children's self-esteem and continue family chaos and parental sense of inadequacy. Don's goal is that of changing unwanted behaviors and learning new behaviors to help children and teens become more responsible, self-sufficient, and self-confident individuals.

The degree of organization, clinical examples, charts, and intervention strategies lend distinctive beauty and effectiveness to this book. This is so helpful for parents reading the book because many of them also have ADD traits themselves. The very organization of Don's book reaches out effectively to these particular parents who need specific structure, order, and step-by-step guidance. This book is an excellent resource for parents who are overwhelmed by details or intimidated by too much informaton. What a gift!

In addition to offering practical, easy-to-understand guidance, the book is equally if not more important because Don's own life circumstances play an integral part of the text. Don grew up having ADHD and raised a daughter who had ADHD. Now, as a therapist in private practice, Don treats ADHD children and their parents. Don's rich and valuable viewpoint of having "walked in others' shoes" is rare and exceptional in a book of this type and allows him to effectively present the materials from three unique perspectives: the ADHD child, the parent, and the therapist. Who better to help than one who has been there and has grown stronger and wiser as a result?

Wild Child is divided into two sections. The first section presents an understanding of the basic nature of ADHD and its diagnosis. The second section deals with therapeutic techniques and treatment. This section is subdivided into two parts that deal with the major practical issues that are essential for proper and effective treatment of children and adolescents. These sections form the heart and soul of the book by informing readers what to do for the child and parents once the diagnosis of ADHD has been made. His understanding of pertinent issues is priceless and his interventions are practical and comprehensive.

Each chapter contains basic rules for children and parents to follow. Ample use of clinical examples illustrates the points made in the text. Practical rubber-meets-the-road guides for parents are given to help their children with familiar and important issues such as aggression, temper tantrums, chores, bedtime difficulties, messy rooms, and getting dressed and ready for school. Breaking curfews, truancy, running away, and substance abuse are some of the many issues addressed in the section on adolescence.

Although *Wild Child* primarily deals with ADHD, it has much broader implications to help treat other important clinical conditions such as oppositional defiant disorder (ODD), anxiety disorders, post-traumatic stress disorder, depression, and much more. Some of these conditions often coexist with ADHD, while some of them masquerade as ADHD due to overlapping clinical features. However, all can be helped substantially by the interventions offered in these core chapters.

Before closing, I want to share the following thoughts about my relationship with Don Mordasini with whom I have worked for several years. Don is an inspiration—consistently positive, affirming, and enthusiastic. However busy, he always makes time to be helpful and readily shares his information and ideas. He is excellent at assessing clinical situations and quickly focuses in on the salient issues. His therapeutic abilities are well honed and he brings into play the skills of a diagnostician, therapist, mentor, teacher, and role model. Don also is able to handle the delicate balance between treating the child or the adolescent while involving the parents in a constructive way. I especially appreciate his follow-up procedures on tough cases and his commitment to helping achieve positive results, which have resulted in remarkable success with a wide variety of patients. He is also quite comfortable and skillful in working with other professionals such as schoolteachers, tutors, counselors, or psychiatrists. He is committed to developing a strong treatment-team alliance. I look forward to continuing my personal and professional relationship with this most talented and special person.

Bruce M. Wermuth, MD
Los Gatos, California

Special Acknowledgments

I wish to thank Hal Zina Bennett for editing *Wild Child*. I imagine it was no easy task for him to edit an ADHD author's manuscript. I know I must have been looking out the window when English grammar was being taught. I thank him for his patience and perseverance.

I also wish to thank Katy Day, typist extraordinaire. How did you get those charts to fit so neatly? And how come all the sentences are in a neat little row?

Introduction

I was in my fifties when I learned that I have attention deficit disorder. Somehow that sounds as though I was late investigating what makes me tick. I was. I was too busy and too successful to slow down and look over my shoulder. When I did glance back, I saw a shadow behind me, so I kept running. Helena, my wife, used to ask me why I did not slow down and take an easier, less stressful job. Each time she said that, I shuddered, not knowing exactly why that suggestion bothered me so much.

I was a professional businessman for twenty years, and during that time my energies were primarily focused on raising a family and building a business. Through trial and error, unaware of my condition, I had learned many coping strategies to manage my life. I was blessed with strong intuition that kept me out of areas of activity where my ADD would have been my downfall. However, the inevitable can only be delayed so long and I met up with myself when I had a nervous breakdown at the age of forty-eight.

During that period I virtually lost my identity. I had been a high achiever in business and I was unable to work any longer. A marriage I treasured for twenty years became unraveled. Divorce and taxes drained the financial security I had built up for retirement. Children I had held and loved every day of my life became frightened of my breakdown, and a distance grew between us. I began a long period of self-loathing. I had identified myself by what I could do and the various hats I wore; none of them fit anymore. I cursed myself as a misfit, weakling, loser, and burden to others.

The period of self-loathing I experienced was the start of my healing, excruciatingly painful though it was. I had come smack up against a deep-rooted belief in my own inadequacy. It was not a new feeling. I had experienced a sense of it from the time I started primary school. It followed me through high school, college, and my career. I had to climb ever-higher mountains to prove my own self-worth.

My identity was in my accomplishments. It was all *out there.* Without my accomplishments I was nothing. I was caught up in the age-old conflict between "doing" and "being." I had to find new ways to be comfortable with myself or perish. I spent the next several years searching for who I really am. I was forced to find my self-worth outside my achievements. I was forced to let go of self-worth concepts based on profession, physical comforts, and material success. I had to stop measuring human worth against any yardstick whatsoever.

Beginning with childhood, I had compared, analyzed, evaluated, interpreted, and reviewed, always comparing myself against others. I always fell far short of the mark: I was not scholastic; I was too clumsy, slow, loud, wild, misbehaving, ad nauseum.

Self-comparison always occurs in the child's mind, and the ADD mind is continually processing such information, sometimes repressing the thoughts, other times entertaining them. *This is the curse of the child's mind and it continues until, as an adult, he or she becomes aware of these thoughts and begins to question their validity.*

When I found out that I had ADD I felt a burden lift from my shoulders. I was able to look at my distorted thinking and begin the true healing process of correcting my own false assumptions of myself. It was my first step toward throwing away the measuring tape. Unfortunately, the healing process does not end with the diagnosis. One tries to throw away the measuring tape only to pick it up again and again. As I began to slow down the mental nonsense, I started to get in touch with my own innate goodness. Nevertheless, the process of reconstructing a view of myself had begun and I was firmly on the path toward self-healing.

This path ultimately brought me to a decision. What was I to do with the rest of my life? As I reflected on this matter, I felt that our planet was seeded with enough stockbrokers that my absence from the profession would not be particularly noticed. I realized that I wanted to use my experience to help others, and since I had crossed the hot coals, I thought I might help others to circumvent them. Thus, I began forging a new career as a psychotherapist.

As a clinician, I believe the most serious harm that can result from undiagnosed and untreated ADD is the painful and devastating loss of self-esteem. With absolutely no malicious intent, parents, teachers, relatives, peers, preachers, television, and the media tend to make it difficult for the ADD child to develop normal self-esteem.

As an insider, so to speak, I have written this book to help parents feel better about their children and to help children feel good about themselves.

My concern is that ADD children learn to trust themselves, feel good about themselves, and have confidence in their worth as unique individuals.

Many parents are concerned about their child's behavior in school and at home: lack of motivation, inability to progress academically with peers, mood swings, temper tantrums, and inability to concentrate. When I was raising my own ADD daughter I was puzzled by these problems. At that time, I had no idea about dealing with these and other ADD issues.

My mission for this period of my life is to help parents and children change unwanted behaviors and learn new behaviors. Although learning new behavior is very important, *the overall goal is to help children become responsible, self-sufficient, self-confident individuals.*

This book is written from three perspectives:

1. The first perspective is that of the ADD child. You have an opportunity to view life through the lens of the ADDer. From this vantage point you can gain an understanding and a fresh appreciation for the challenges an ADD child faces.
2. The second perspective is that of the parent (myself) working with a very demanding ADD child, caught up with my own bewilderment, frustration, and occasional sense of helplessness.
3. The third perspective is from the vantage point of a clinician. This perspective is the hand holding, tutoring, and the explaining part, offering new ways to help your child. I have tried to be very careful to take you slowly, step by step, through each chapter so that you build upon your own knowledge and experience. This allows you to build confidence in your ability to help your child develop a solid sense of self as he or she learns new constructive behaviors with your guidance.

I no longer run from my shadow. We are one. Thank God! The difficulties I experienced as I faced myself gave me a deeper appreciation of who I really am. Deep inside me I found a love for humankind, and, even more wonderful than that, I discovered how I could use my experiences to help others. To be able to follow my bliss, as the great mythologist Joseph Campbell would say, is a very great gift indeed!

PART I: DEVELOPING UNDERSTANDING

Chapter 1

My Struggle As a Parent

I am amazed, me thinks, and lose my way
Among the thorns and dangers of this world.

Shakespeare
King John III

My story begins approximately thirty years ago when I first met Manuela. She was the healthy, happy, rosy-cheeked three-year-old daughter of my fiancée, Helena. Manuela lived in a storybook town, high in the Austrian Alps, in a village that skiers flocked to from all over the world. Kitzbuehel, the renowned skiing and après-ski life village, had called to me as well.

I was practicing sitzmarks in the snow during *Fasching,* a time of carnival that lasts approximately three weeks, until the eve of *Ashen Mittwoch* (Ash Wednesday) at which time everyone nurses their hangovers and catches up on sleep. During this period of reveling, I met Helena, whom I married a few months later.

My first images of Manuela were in the city garden where she would prance about picking flowers. She loved flowers. She would pick them and give them to relatives, friends, and her mother. Manuela was extremely gregarious. Frequently, I would ask where Manuela was; the most common answer was that she was having a *kaffee klatsch* with one of the neighbors. When she brought flowers to the neighbors they offered her tea, milk, and sometimes sweets. She would chat away, seated in a chair and swinging her legs, while carrying on a very adult conversation. Those are my fondest memories of this beautiful alpine child with big red cheeks who was loved by everyone who knew her.

Shortly after Helena and I married, we moved to Langen, a suburb of Frankfurt, where I had secured work that would support us. I dearly missed the healthy, vigorous climate of the Alps and we returned frequently, as time would allow. Manuela continued winning the hearts of the adults in the apartment building we moved to, continuing her grand tradition of *kaffee klatsches* purchased with gifts of flowers. City life was different in that Helena was concerned that Manuela sometimes took flowers from the front of cafés and small gardens, but no one seemed to mind.

A few months later, Helena became pregnant with Beate. I stayed in Langen, commuting to Frankfurt for work, while Helena and Manuela moved to Kitzbuehel to be with her family during the later stages of her pregnancy. I visited frequently. However, when my young family was ready to move to Langen to be with me, we encountered problems with passports. I was American; Beate was also American born on foreign soil. Helena was Austrian and was unable to place Beate on her passport, which was the customary procedure when newborn children traveled from one country to another with their parents. It took time for me to register Beate's birth at the embassy, take pictures, and have a passport issued in her name. When passports were finally straightened out, my family arrived in Germany. I enjoyed the girls and my new family life began. Manuela was very protective of Beate; she played second mother very well. The next year was an idyllic one.

My career was not flourishing in Frankfurt, so I moved with the family from Langen to the United States, settling in San Francisco near relatives and friends where I began my career as a stockbroker.

Manuela was of preschool age, so we enrolled her in German class on Saturdays. I remembered how much effort I had put into learning German and thought it would be wonderful for her to grow up bilingual.

The first red flags began to appear. We started receiving confusing reports from her teachers. They said she was a delightful child and very friendly. When she read out loud she read as well as any of the children in the class but she did not seem to learn anything new, and they questioned whether she understood what she was reading.

One day I came home from work and noticed the children playing outside our apartment were calling Manuela "Susie." I asked

Manuela why they were calling her that and she said that she did not know how to tell them her name because she could not tell them in English. At that moment I realized it was important for us to speak English at home so that Manuela would not be at a disadvantage when she started regular school.

I had assumed children would grow up bilingual if left to themselves in the proper environment which is not necessarily so. They may speak both languages, but if they do not have average learning skills, their knowledge of language can handicap them. By this time it was clear that Manuela was not making progress with her class in German school.

We began speaking English at home and Manuela learned it quickly. I began to see that there were different ways to learn but it did not occur to me that she might have trouble in a structured academic environment. Since she was speaking English so well the issue of learning fell to the back of my mind. Before long it was time to enroll Manuela in the first grade. I wanted to enroll her in a Catholic school but was told that she was not mature enough to manage the curriculum. I was quite surprised and made a big fuss about this to no avail.

Manuela attended public school at a time when I was very busy building my career. I assumed she would be fine and paid little attention to school activities. Near her completion of the first grade, Manuela's teacher told us she was not doing well. When I saw the report cards I was extremely upset. If something was not done immediately, she was destined to be held back. I hired a tutor and her grades improved. Following that experience, I decided to monitor her progress more carefully.

The teacher said that when Manuela was left alone she had trouble learning. I chalked this up to Manuela socializing at inappropriate times. I had no idea that she might not be able to concentrate as well as the other children, or that she was at a disadvantage in any way. The fact that she did better with tutors strengthened my hypothesis that they probably did not allow distracting conversation. They were apparently providing a tight structure for her and the more personal teaching was effective because they could work closely with her distractibility and motivate her.

At that time, I assumed all children could learn in a school environment unless they were of borderline intelligence. I knew children had to put in varying degrees of effort to master a subject, but I thought those children who could not keep pace with their peers were lazy or goof-offs. Less was known about attention deficit disorder thirty years ago. I only wish someone had approached me with the information that Manuela had ADD.

By the time Manuela reached third grade, she was really struggling. This time her social behavior was becoming a problem. She was difficult to manage in class; she was also making friends with other children who had behavior problems.

I thought she was deliberately not working in school. I came from a stern family and was influenced by the ideas I inherited from my parents. Like my parents, I used stern measures in my efforts to motivate Manuela, which created a lot of misunderstanding. A gap grew between us that we never really breached until she became an adult.

I was in a dilemma. What to do? The "Big Struggle" to get your child to do what he or she does not want to do, or does not have the capacity to do, can be frustrating, to say the least. I was bewildered and worn out from cajoling, pleading, punishing, rewarding, and nagging. Nothing I did seemed to work. Unbeknownst to me, I was undermining Manuela's fragile sense of self-esteem. She acquired my perception of her as inadequate and lazy; her self-confidence spiraled downward. The seeds were sown for her to dislike herself. Low self-esteem had found fertile breeding grounds.

Today, I believe most of the problems our young people encounter stem from their inability to accept and love themselves. Many years passed, however, before this became entirely clear to me in my own family. Both Helena and I thought that if we loved our children enough they would learn love. We showed our love in many ways and were able to give them material comforts that were beyond the reach of many families.

I understand very clearly now that the parents' perception of giving love is not necessarily adequate for the child to feel loved. When a child believes he or she is not loved, he or she experiences the pain of rejection and frequently manifests this pain as misbehavior.

Helena had grown up in Austria and attended school during World War II. At that time, most European children were deprived of the basic necessities. Food was scarce and starvation was not infrequent. She faced austerities that are unknown to us today. As with many Europeans, Helena thought the United States was a land of equal opportunity for all and could not understand why her daughter so casually dismissed all our efforts to get her a basic education. She was at a complete loss to understand how Manuela could throw away such golden opportunities. I was in full agreement with my wife's sentiments. I also thought our situation was unique. I did not know other parents were letting go of future dreams for their children as they wrestled with the challenges their children faced. We were also letting go of our belief that a combination of love and money could cure anything. I had no way of comprehending that Manuela simply wanted salve for her wounds. I did not even understand that she was wounded.

Even further from my mind was the thought that she might have a hypersensitive nervous system that made her more sensitive to her environment, and that studying, remembering, and paying attention were slightly beyond her grasp without professional support.

Years slipped by as Helena and I cajoled, pushed, threatened, harassed, and struggled with Manuela to get passing grades in school. Somehow we all muddled through the next few years. Our problems did not end with poor academic performance. Manuela became belligerent at home, acted out her frustrations on Beate and her youngest sister, Monika, our last addition to the family, and became very difficult to live with.

One insight stood out among all the thoughts I had at the time. We were driving to my mother's house for a Sunday visit and I remarked to Helena that it was more difficult for Beate and Monika, our other two children, to do something wrong than it was for Manuela to do something right. This thought was an epiphany for me and I wondered how God could do this to a child. I remember thinking that this was unfair, and it was the first glimpse of compassion I had for Manuela in a long time.

I soon found out that my not-quite seventh grader was using marijuana and drinking alcohol. I was jolted by the realization that my daughter was using drugs. I thought by lecturing her and grounding her she would be motivated to make better choices. Instead, it only served to separate us further. More problems developed as Manuela found support from other children like herself who had dropped out of mainstream culture.

Throughout this trying time, it never occurred to me that she might be suffering from a known mental disorder. Teachers, friends, colleagues, neighbors, and family, all of whom knew of our problems with Manuela, never suggested that we might consider a psychological evaluation or testing. The evidence is so overwhelming to me today that it seems inconceivable that I did not think of this at the time. But it simply never occurred to me. I was so caught up in the daily clashing of egos that I could not step back and see the larger picture.

What had happened to the beautiful child I had first met at Kitzbuehel, the loving flower child who had taken such delight in pleasing the people who loved her? I cursed the United States that somehow had brought out the worst in my daughter. Beate and Monika were so easy to be with. Why was Manuela so difficult? I would look at the pictures of Manuela in our Austrian garden as she happily picked flowers and gave them to us. It was difficult to believe how much she had changed.

Years later, when Manuela sought treatment as an adult, the pieces fell together. With the help of my friend, Dr. Phil Kavanaugh, who diagnosed ADD in me, we were finally able to diagnose my daughter and obtain relief for her as well.

As I reflected on Manuela's struggles, I realized that I learned a lot from my experiences with her that should be shared with others facing similar problems. One of the gifts of those years is the fact that I am able to understand the thoughts, emotions, and interactional processes other parents experience with their ADD children. In addition to that, I hopefully understand more clearly how the child feels. Also, I am now able to understand my own early years a little better and realize why I acted the way I did as a hyperactive child.

Hopefully, our greatest challenges in life can be passed along to others as lessons and insights to make their lives a little easier. That awareness, so many years after my own children have grown into adulthood, is what I pass along to parents and children with whom I now work. Some of the key ideas are described in the following chapters.

Chapter 2

What My Personal Experience Has Taught Me

Experience is the name everyone gives to their mistakes.

Oscar Wilde
Lady Windermere's Fan

PARENTAL RIGIDNESS

Perhaps the most important lesson I learned through my struggles with Manuela is that children who act out at home and in school are not just lazy, stupid, or goof-offs. My own rigidness on this point probably prevented me from seeking reasons for my daughter's behavior.

Parental rigidness prevents children from getting the help they need. Frequently, one parent will want to explore treatment and the other will resist it. One of my frustrations today is seeing children denied treatment because the more rigid parent has the louder voice and insists the child is simply lazy or unappreciative. This rigidness only exaggerates the problem, further alienating the child, lowering his or her* sense of self-worth, and escalating the unwanted behavior.

---

*Every attempt has been made to keep the text gender neutral. In instances where changes would result in awkward format, the masculine pronouns have been retained.

CAUSE-EFFECT BEHAVIOR

I also learned that all behaviors make sense to the child. Although I could not understand why Manuela did the things she did, her behavior made perfect sense to her.

Many parents do not understand why their child is belligerent, obstinate, noncooperative, and so forth. I ask them why they think their child will not study, disobeys them, and engages in sabotaging behavior. I tell them that all reactions make sense. I point out, usually with the help of the child, that a refusal to study might be because the child does not understand the assignment, or perhaps the assignment appears too long and overwhelming. The obstinate child sometimes freezes because he does not want to make a mistake or look stupid. Sabotaging behavior is "getting even" behavior. The child, who feels unfairly treated because of loss of privileges or ridiculing, finds a way to release these pent-up frustrations. As I discuss cause-effect behavior and use examples from their child's actions that make sense to them, adults begin to understand that their child does have specific motives for acting out. Parents may have trouble following the logic of their children or accepting that their own best intentions create problems for them. However, some acknowledgment of that process, with all its potential for conflict, frequently paves the way for parents and children to develop a more constructive relationship.

EMOTIONAL ENMESHMENT

I learned that my emotional distress and frustration as a parent prevented me from thinking rationally and acting like an adult. Instead, I often found myself tangling emotionally with my child, reduced to her level of immaturity. Instead of being the one who stood for reason, stability, and trust, I often abandoned Manuela emotionally because my behavior mirrored hers.

Most parents I meet in my practice are emotionally enmeshed with their children, just as I once was. In fact, this is one of the main reasons parents seek professional help. I help them learn new ways to interact with their children. The help of a professional who is not emotionally involved can focus each family member's attention on problem solving, rather than escalating the words and actions that are causing the problem.

LOSS OF SELF-ESTEEM

Children are like sponges and cannot help but take in the judgments of parents, family, peers, and teachers. The most important influences for developing an adequate sense of self are in the child's home. The child's ability to develop self-confidence and a sense of self-worth must be given top priority *even above getting good grades at school!*

Many of the children I work with feel their parents do not love them. They cite the punishment and the angry way their parents behave toward them. These children believe that something is wrong with them that makes them "bad," and causes the parents' behavior. These children believe that they are lazy or stupid or cannot learn or remember to do things correctly. They do not understand that they have ADD and, therefore, tasks that are easy for their siblings are frequently very difficult for them. Without this understanding they think negatively of themselves, particularly if the child/parent emotional struggle is intense. Lacking self-esteem and the confidence to do things that will please their parents, they may seek a very negative form of "power," gained by outraging or angering their parents. A cycle builds in which the parents fail to esteem the ADD child because of these dynamics and the child loses confidence in his ability to manage tasks he should be mastering.

A SENSE OF PERSPECTIVE/NEW LEARNING

Because of my emotional enmeshment and the daily clashing of egos, I was unable to step back and consider new ways to deal with Manuela's and my own problem. I did not realize that my interventions were causing Manuela's reactions. I was stuck in old habits, old ways of behaving. I needed to learn new skills and stop expecting my daughter to do most of the work. In a sense, I needed new learning as a way to keep the "big picture" of Manuela's future in mind.

Parents need to learn how to help their children with school and behavior problems. It can be difficult for parents to let go of judgments, expectations, and negative emotional enmeshment. Minimally, adults need to be aware of their own emotional reactions so that they can interact with their child from a rational, thoughtful perspective. The ideal occurs when the parent is able to uphold a model for the child to follow. The information discussed in the next several chapters deals with this issue.

THE POWER STRUGGLE

One of the most important lessons I learned involved the dilemma of getting lost in the power struggle between my daughter and me. The struggle for control is a very basic dynamic, one that thwarts most parents' attempts to help their children.

Who is in charge? That's a key question. If parents do not establish dominance over the child, the chances are that nothing will change and the child will get his or her own way. A mature and rational individual is required to steer the relationship and the child in a positive direction. The problem with most parents who dominate their ADD child is that they take total control and the child is not able to participate in working out compromises or cocreating solutions. This places the child in a position of helplessness, enduring whatever fairness or unfairness the parents dispense. Because most parents of ADD children need to build new parenting skills, they often react emotionally to the child by initially overlooking behavior that needs to be addressed and severely punishing smaller transgressions as their frustration mounts. Thrust into a helpless position, resentment and anger build in the child. He or she struggles against helplessness both passively (not obeying parents, not studying, etc.) and aggressively (in shouting matches, tantrums, and various acting-out behaviors). The problem is that when the child is old enough to take control, usually as a teenager, the parent becomes virtually helpless and so the roles are reversed. We see this throughout our country where youths gather, use illicit drugs, have skirmishes with the law, destroy property, and often begin exploring their sexuality. Many parents then fall into the previous behavior of their children, passively giving up on them as helpless cases or striking out at them with verbal or even physical abuse.

I frequently encounter families where the young child is in charge. In such cases the parents are passive, or are afraid of angering the child who is out of control, for fear of engaging the child's rage and making things worse. Sometimes these parents are burned out from the continuous struggle, so they just give up or give in. Other times, alcoholism or emotional problems interfere with the adult's ability to parent the child. The child throws temper tantrums, is disrespectful to parents, hits siblings and parents, and, in general, dominates the family as he or she pleases. ADD children need structure in the household because they lack sufficient structure within themselves. Additionally, they instinctively know that they have behavior problems and do not have the resources to create a safe and nurturing family system themselves. Although they do not reveal this to their parents and probably cannot express it themselves, they definitely need safety and structure that they cannot provide on their own. The ADD child does not have the maturity to be in control of the family, yet this frequently happens. Out of fear of being dominated, the child seeks control that is not really wanted. These children fear facing their own problems that they believe are unsolvable. And they fear change because that means facing the unknown that they feel ill equipped to handle.

The power struggle for family dominance and the power struggle to gain a voice in the parent-dominated system continue in full force at a heavy cost to both parties.

The key to getting your child to behave in an age-appropriate manner is cooperation. Developing cooperation between parent and child, setting goals, and communicating are important components of working together. The parents need to be in control of the child to allow this to take place. The job is to put down the general's hat and take up the conflict resolution banner. I spend most of my therapy hours coaching parents and children to avoid the pitfalls of the Big Struggle.

When parents find themselves constantly struggling with their children, it can seem to them that their present difficulties will never end. Time moves slowly from season to season. It is difficult for them to see the future; it appears so distant, so far away. Frequently, time itself seems to stand still as they set limit after limit that their children oppose. However, children do grow up and the results of good work bear fruit. I have had many children tell me that they fought their parents during their younger years and are thankful for the safety and structure that was provided them at that time. Parents, too, tell me of their frustrations and the trembling they sometimes experience while under attack. The appreciation sometimes comes many years after the struggle has ended, but it comes. On the other hand, I have had countless parents thank me for the changes they see in their children as they receive direction and support from other professionals or me.

Parents who have been struggling on their own, without help or guidance, find that the task becomes easier and both they and their children get along better when they at last get professional help. Although the children do not always acknowledge it, parents find relief and appreciation for their efforts resulting in positive change long before their children are grown.

The last holdout is the child's denial that anything has changed, even when it is quite clear that it has. Just recently, I was working with a four-member family. Brent, ten years old, informed me that he had not experienced any changes since starting therapy and medication for ADD. His parents recounted how he was doing his homework assignments and turning them in on time. His teacher allowed him to be "class monitor" for the week because of his much improved school performance. At home he was obeying his parents and completing his chores. His parents were beaming with pride at their son while he sat in my office, sketching pictures, telling me that he was the same kid.

While I learned many lessons from my personal experience with my daughter, as well as by reflecting on my own childhood, I believe the previous discussion summarizes the key ideas most parents find helpful.

The remainder of this book discusses ways to develop new interaction patterns to effectively deal with the problems mentioned throughout this chapter. The techniques discussed have come from my personal and clinical experience as a therapist. The ideas and techniques put forth are the same ones I use in therapy sessions.

Chapter 3

Attention Deficit Disorder
from the Inside Out

There is nothing in this world constant but inconstancy.

Jonathan Swift
The Battle of the Books

WHAT IS ATTENTION DEFICIT
(HYPERACTIVITY) DISORDER?

As a child I experienced my world through the perspective of what today we call "attention deficit hyperactivity disorder." My perception, of course, was my reality. To me, it was what was actually happening out there; it was my truth. What I thought people thought about me, what I thought my parents felt about me, particularly what I thought about myself, was simply true. It never occurred to me that other people might experience life differently. It never occurred to me that my parents' thoughts about me were different from what I believed they were.

It is sometimes difficult for parents to understand why their children do what they do. This is particularly true when children do not conform to their parents' expectations. Parents fall into this trap so easily. If a child has ADD, their behavior is even more difficult for parents to understand. It takes most of us a long time to realize that perception, whether it is ours or other people's, is not the same as reality. We each create our unique experiences of our world. This is simply a fact of human life.

In an effort to clearly communicate what an ADD person might experience, I decided to share a few stories from my childhood. After each of the following vignettes is a clinical explanation of the particular ADD trait that behavior would fall under.

I DO NOT REMEMBER!

I remember sitting in class at Catholic school and making up a calendar in February or March, counting the school days left until summer vacation. I also counted the number of actual weekdays until the bell for freedom struck. Each school day I would cross out another day and reduce my number by one. As the number of days before summer vacation dropped below sixty, I would begin to get really excited. I had two lists: the list of school days, which was shorter, and the list of counting a week as seven days, which was longer. I always paid strict attention to the shorter list but felt a little queasy inside, as though I was cheating myself. Once in a while I would announce to a playmate that there were only seventy-eight days of school remaining, exclusive of weekends and holidays. I never could understand their lack of enthusiasm or excitement about this startling tidbit of information.

When I got into trouble, particularly if there were two or fewer school months remaining, it was not stressful to me because I knew I would soon be liberated. I would think, "They can't punish me because in a short time it won't mean anything."

I was able to focus on this information very well. I knew the numbers by heart and could easily do all the calculations quickly in my mind. Somehow I was not able to carry that focus to academic subjects. The teacher would be talking and I would "come to," suddenly realizing I had missed a lot of information. I drifted easily. Other times, I knew something important was being discussed and would try my hardest to pay attention. But then I would just drift away and find myself not listening to the teacher. I was extremely motivated in drawing up my chart of school days; therefore, I was able to hyper-focus on this information. School subjects did not motivate me enough to hold my attention. Many parents become confused when they see their child hyper-focus or "get lost" in a high stimulation activity and believe that the child should be able to apply the same focus to academic subjects. ADD children are not usually able to do this. Unless the stimulation is great or the motivation very high, they lose their concentration.

If we had to plan a project that required homework and in-class work over a period of time, I felt confused and frightened because I did not know how to begin or continue whatever I might start. I felt completely overwhelmed, which only increased my anxiety and confusion.

I honestly do not ever remember getting many homework assignments. If I got them I just dashed them off to get it over with. I remember my dad calling me a liar because I did not have homework while my brother, three years my junior, would bring home one or two hours of work from the same school. Dad would make me copy a page from the encyclopedia if I did not have homework. I thought he was a bully and I hated him for this. The next day I would show up without homework again, only to continue transcribing the encyclopedia. I think my dislike of the encyclopedia today stems from this experience.

I also thought the kids who received good grades were really smart. Certainly much smarter than I was! I did not particularly like most of the kids who received good grades. I was also puzzled at how they could stretch out and complicate homework assignments that I thought were relatively simple. Additionally, I never remembered hearing the teacher talk about half the assignments that my peers reported. It was as if we lived in different worlds. In a way, I suppose, we really did.

INATTENTIVENESS

Most children are selectively inattentive and this is to be expected. However, the ADD child's mind wanders relentlessly. He or she has trouble focusing on homework, listening to instructions, following instructions, paying attention in class, and remembering parents' advice. This child daydreams constantly. The short attention span of this child means he or she gets bored easily, tunes out conversations, and appears never to be fully present mentally. Forgetfulness is another characteristic of this child. These children will not remember what you tell them, even moments after your most impassioned scolding. They misplace objects, leave completed homework assignments at home, and will generally drive you crazy with their apparent inattentiveness.

They may engage in a lot of activity yet accomplish little or nothing. They may begin projects enthusiastically but fail to follow through. You may notice some correlation between high interest activities and ability to hold attention with them, particularly in certain play situations. Although motivation does play a role, the problem is that the child's head is on a swivel. Everything seems to call for the child's attention, and so he or she finds it difficult to give full attention to any one thing.

As strange as it seems, this child also has the ability to hyperfocus, becoming involved in computer games for hours at a time, or getting completely lost in athletic activities. While this may seem to be a contradiction, it is not. Most theorists believe the ability to "lock on" and get lost in an activity is an expression of the brain's desire to calm itself. As mentioned above, many parents think that if their child can focus on Nintendo for hours but cannot sit still for homework then that child must be lazy or just plain obstinate. It is important to recognize that total immersion in a highly motivated activity, such as computer games, does not rule out the possibility that the child has ADD.

My Feelings Are Hurt

I was a very sensitive child. My parents praised my younger brother, Jerry, who was always an excellent student. They doted on my sister, Gail, who was ten years my junior. While they doted on Gail and gloated about Jerry, nothing much was said about me, except maybe that I drank too much milk, and water was cheaper. I was also informed that clothes were expensive and I wore mine out much faster than my brother. I grew up with the perception that I was a nuisance to my whole family.

When I was in the fifth grade I delivered daily newspapers. I did this for two years. I did not want to ask my parents for money; I did not want to be dependent upon them. Finally, they threatened to take my paper route away because my grades were so poor. I remember them telling my school principal, Sister De Sales, that "Donny doesn't have to work, so we will take his job away if it will improve his grades." My mother added, "We are not like some of the other families whose children have to work." The *"have to"* got special emphasis. In the eighth grade I sold newspapers on San Francisco street corners. A good day meant I earned a dollar.

I never asked my parents for anything. I did not want to experience the feeling of being disappointed and rejected if they refused. One Christmas I was told that money was tight so each child would get a dollar for each year of age. I was about eleven so I would be given eleven dollars. I was given a Sears catalog and told to pick out my presents. Gail was only three so this rule could not apply to her. My brother was only six so that would not be enough money for him. I remember being unable to experience my disappointment and hurt. Instead, I tried to be cheerful. *I knew I was in the way. I vowed never to ask anybody for anything for the rest of my life.*

Feeling unappreciated or unloved is very difficult. I did not know anything different, of course. But I did recognize that I was not treated the same as other kids. I did not get as much homework as the other kids did. I never thought to ask why. I did not get good grades because I was not smart. Dad would sometimes say, "Donny is strong. He'll make a good truck driver." If I gave it any thought at all, I would probably have agreed with my father's appraisal. I did not like to think of myself as a beast of burden. But then, I did not like to think about myself at all! It was just too depressing.

HYPERSENSITIVITY

ADD children appear to be more sensitive than their peers are. This sensitivity can manifest in many different ways. The child frequently has a "thin skin," and is more easily wounded emotionally. He or she will tend to personalize transactions among peers and elders that are neutral. It would not be unusual to hear such a child say, "That person is staring at me," or, "That person doesn't like me. I can tell!" This child will take offense easily, cry readily, be cranky, moody, or withdraw quickly. The ADD child is subject to wide mood swings. One moment everything is fine, the next moment a crisis has emerged.

These children fight a lot with their siblings. Simple exchanges turn into bruised feelings. Shouting and screaming may occur. One minute this child is playing nicely, the next he or she is in a fight.

The ADD child has a low frustration tolerance. Environment, friends, parents, and siblings need to be a certain way or emotions are aroused. This child is very moody. Change is difficult for him or her. Because of this sensitivity, the ADD child often lives on an emotional roller coaster, up and seemingly in high spirits one moment, in a pit of gloomy despair the next.

In addition to emotional sensitivity, ADD children feel different from their peers. They look at others and think of themselves as deficient because they cannot be like them. Not understanding their unique nervous system, and therefore having a difficult way of being in the world, they get down on themselves easily. They feel inadequate, judge themselves unfairly, and are unable to soothe these uncomfortable and even painful feelings. Unfortunately, adults (parents, relatives, neighbors, and sometimes teachers) unknowingly contribute to ADD children's feelings of low self-esteem. Any kind of conflict with adults around them reinforces these feelings of inadequacy.

This child tends to act out these sensitive feelings. Acting out is one of the more serious problems we encounter with ADD children. That is, rather than telling another person that they are confused or upset, they will attempt to discharge their feelings through their actions. These actions are often chaotic, even to the child. They usually have a negative effect on other people. Young people will withdraw, become uncommunicative, engage in passive-aggressive behavior, or react aggressively and chaotically. The aggressive child is frequently angry, spiteful, and will strike out at others, sometimes indiscriminately.

If these problems are not addressed by the teen years—that is, if the teen does not learn how to soothe his own feelings or express them in a constructive way, in order to feel good about himself— problems can escalate exponentially. The use of illicit drugs or alcohol, sexual acting out, and problems with the law can follow.

Hypersensitivity tends to be a problem with ADD children, adolescents, and adults. The thin skin remains that way until the ADDer learns to take greater control over his own perceptions, thoughts, and emotions.

Donny Can't Sit Still

As a child, I was a first-class fidgeter. I could not sit still. One day my mother and I paid a visit to the principal's office to discuss this problem. No one could figure out why I squirmed so much. The principal asked me if my shoes were too tight, or if my clothing was uncomfortable. I answered, "No." Not only did I fidget, but also I made noises that I was not aware of. No solution was found.

I had boundless energy. I loved to wrestle. In the eighth grade, a friend of mine would visit me on Friday nights when my parents went to the drive-in movies with the rest of the children. I was allowed to stay home because I thought I was too grown up to watch a movie with my siblings and I was starting to form important teenage peer relationships. I was not allowed in the living room, except for those special occasions when relatives or guests were invited to the house. This was a very strict rule that all of us had to follow. My friend, Joey, would walk about two miles to visit me because my family had a television and few others in the neighborhood did. I would see Joey Friday afternoons and say, "Hey, Joey, why don't you come over and watch some television tonight?" Before I would let Joey watch television, though, I put him through the following ordeal: We would remove all the furniture from the living room, piece by piece, including the sofa, to prepare the wrestling arena. Then the wrestling would begin. We would have three matches. A match was over when one of us would give up. I was a bit stronger than Joey, which meant he had to get beaten three times. I loved it. It was so much fun! When the wrestling matches were over, we carefully placed each piece of furniture back in its original position and then watched television in another room. My mother was very particular about having a clean house. If she had known what I had done she would have been furious.

I remember another occasion that was humorous. I was older and my parents had a nice cabin in the country about a two-hour drive from San Francisco. We never used it off-season except to prepare it for the summer season. One day, when I was in my late teens, I had the bright idea to take my friends to the cabin during the winter. About six of us went to the cabin, girls included.

The cabin had beautiful solid wood rafters that spanned the room. We went into the cabin and before long were using the couches like trampolines to jump to the rafters and swing from them like monkeys. I never enjoyed myself so much. A few months later I went with my dad to help prepare the cabin for summer. We climbed a ladder to the attic, which was just above the rafters. Dad suddenly turned to me and said, "Look at all those fingerprints in the dust along the rafters. How in the world could they ever get there?" I told him I had no idea.

HYPERACTIVITY (ADHD TRAIT)

The primary difference between the attention deficit disorder child (ADD) and the attention deficit hyperactivity child (ADHD) is that the ADHD child exhibits the traits of impulsiveness and hyperactivity that the ADD child does not.

The basic problem with the hyperactive child is that he or she has difficulty controlling behavior. The ADHD child is always on the move, has trouble sitting still, fidgets, squirms, and giggles. This child is easily over-stimulated. Escalation of activity quickly follows what others might regard as a simple, transient action. A water gun fight turns into a war with hoses and buckets of water. Simple touching turns into a wrestling match. Once revved up, this child has trouble slowing down or stopping.

In the classroom, the child is out of his or her seat, has to go to the bathroom, playfully tries to get others in trouble, and gets bored when not stimulated. The child has trouble playing alone and needs physical activity to work off high energy. This child is a jet engine. He or she has a fast acceleration, a high plateau, and trouble coming down.

ADHD children may have a diminished need for sleep and show motor restlessness in bed (kick covers off). They might be excessive talkers and have difficulty listening as words pour from their mouths.

In places where being still is appropriate behavior, such as attending school or church, this child frequently has trouble. Being in a group situation where he or she must take turns requires patience. This hyper-agitation usually renders these types of experiences beyond the child's capacity.

Obeying parents is a challenge when this child is on the run. The child has trouble following orders when wrapped up in activity. He or she is late to dinner, last to come in the house after play, and, when a little older, is frequently gone from the house seeking stimulation elsewhere. Home is boring to this child, who frequently complains there is nothing to do.

Why Won't the Others Follow Me?

When I was about ten years old, I thought of myself as Tarzan, King of the Apes. I read all the comic books and dreamed about living in the jungle, swinging from trees with my monkeys. One day, I decided to lead a band of young Tarzans through the treacherous jungle. We ran and jumped over obstacles, becoming more and more daring as we continued playing. The final challenge was to make a huge jump from the railing of our neighbor's house, catch the lip of their first story patio, walk hand-over-hand to the other side, and then jump down. Nobody wanted to do it. I told them I would go first and demonstrate the maneuver but they all refused, saying it could not be done. I figured they all were afraid and could never make it alone in the jungle. I stood balanced on the railing, swinging my arms to get upward momentum without losing my balance. Finally, I flung myself skyward and caught the edge of the patio that was smooth with dust. For a brief moment I knew Tarzan had performed the impossible task and was elated. But as my body swung parallel with the decking, driven by my momentum, I lost my grip. I landed on my head and could not move. I experienced agonizing pain and was carried into the house, where Aunt Rita nursed me. She asked me, "Who do you think you are, Tarzan?" That hurt as much as the pain in my head!

I was always a risk taker. Another time I was with some friends and saw a rope hanging down from a tree. The branch was over the middle of a dry creekbed. It took about an hour for us to grab the rope with branches we held, and get it to the bank of the creek. Nobody wanted to try to swing. They were afraid that the rope might be too weak or the branch not strong enough to support our weight. I could not believe their fearful arguments. The image of swinging high over the creek was too exciting to be passed up. I grabbed the rope and swung high over the creek. However, as the rope and I started the return trip the branch broke and I came crashing down into the dry creekbed. The fall stunned me.

My mother told me years later that whenever the kids knocked on the door and said, "Donny is hurt," she never knew whether to expect me to be dead or alive. Fortunately, the hospital emergency room was not far from where we lived!

IMPULSIVENESS (ADHD TRAIT)

Hyperactivity and impulsiveness usually occur together. Both are common traits of the ADHD child.

For the impulsive child, a thought almost instantly turns into action. There is barely a second between thought and response. If someone points out to an ADHD child that there is risk, or that his or her decision or choice is not a good one, the desire to act out the action is so strong that the prevailing arguments are ignored. The impulsive child runs across the street without looking for traffic, blurts out answers in class, interrupts others, and takes over games without thinking.

This child is a poor decision maker and has difficulty reflecting on the eventual outcome of the choices he or she makes. For the ADHD child, a thought becomes a desire that needs gratification. The consequences of this impulsiveness are that a lot of mistakes are made.

In a conversation, these children can barely restrain themselves from interrupting others. They feel a great urgency to spill out the contents of their minds. Because they have trouble listening to the needs of others, they may tend to be bossy and think that everyone should do what they want to. Impatience is the hallmark of these children. They have minimal planning ability, if any. Long-term school projects are difficult. As they grow older, they like immediate answers and solutions to problems, no matter how complex they may be.

This child is like the classic gunfighter of the Old West. Shoot first and ask questions later. Never mind that a few innocents are killed along the way!

PEER RELATIONSHIPS

Some children with ADD are more self-absorbed than their peers are. They lack a certain degree of "other" awareness. The more a child is "pulled into himself or herself " the more he or she is going to miss subtle nonverbal cues that other children pick up on naturally. Many ADD children are overwhelmed by their own hyperactivity and impulsiveness to a point that they have trouble being present with other people at all. Thus, social contact can be a problem for both the ADD and ADHD child. Making friends and playing with others becomes a challenge to these children, but we should not forget that it is a challenge they need to overcome.

Because of their low opinions of themselves, these children may find it difficult to accept blame. Blame means there is something wrong with them, and their perception is that they have to be right all the time. They will not admit to making a mistake even when the truth is staring them in the face. The consequences are grave; other children do not like to play with them because they do not "play fair."

It is not unusual for their moodiness and/or irritability to interfere with their play activities. Children do not like to play with "babies," that is, other children who cannot handle their emotions. Most children can be painfully critical of their playmates. ADD children are often the targets of their peers' criticisms and insults.

Frequently, ADD children do not know the unwritten rules of play activities, such as sharing play objects, taking turns in a game, not "hogging" the ball, not crying if they do not get their way, and so forth. These children need to be coached in play, paying particular attention to learning and respecting rules. Playing with a single companion is simpler than playing with a group of children for these kids. Similarly, playing with younger children, who are less sophisticated in the subtleties of play, frequently works for them, in part because the ADD child can control younger children.

Even when ADD children improve their play skills, their peers may remember them as they were and be reluctant to have anything to do with them.

Notes

The previous discussion concludes the cluster of behaviors I see most frequently in ADD and ADHD children. It is presented here as an outline for you to increase your awareness so that a common language is in place to use as we move ahead. It is definitely not meant to be a diagnostic tool and should not be used for these purposes.

For purposes of simplicity I will be referring to both ADD and ADHD children as ADD or attention deficit kids.

SOME FREQUENTLY ASKED QUESTIONS

Q. Does attention deficit disorder affect girls and boys equally?

A. Girls tend to be less hyper. Approximately 80 percent of girls are diagnosed with inattentiveness without the hyperactivity frequently seen in boys (ADD). Boys, on the other hand, tend to exhibit inattention as well as hyperactivity and impulsiveness

(ADHD). Girls who did not have hyperactivity, which is easily noticed, have presented a problem in the past because their inattentiveness tended to be overlooked. Or it was assumed by teachers and parents to be a sign of laziness, lack of intelligence, or daydreaming.

Q. Does this mean that there are different diagnostic types of ADD?
A. Yes, the American Psychiatric Association breaks down ADD into three types:

1. Attention deficit disorder, predominantly inattentive type.
2. Attention deficit hyperactivity disorder, predominantly hyperactive-impulsive type.
3. Attention deficit hyperactivity disorder, combined type.

Q. If my child exhibits some ADD traits, does this mean he needs to be treated for attention deficit disorder?
A. No, children may experience some ADD symptoms for a number of reasons. Frequently children with depression and/or anxiety disorders will be disruptive, act out excessively, and have difficulty paying attention. Any child can experience some of these traits to varying degrees. This in no way suggests that they may have ADD. The following example illustrates this point.

Recently, I interviewed a young adult who complained of ADD symptoms. On the surface it appeared he might indeed have attention deficit disorder. He changed jobs frequently, was bored easily, changed residences several times a year, and had a history of trouble maintaining stable relationships. As I evaluated him, I found that his problems were caused by difficulties he experienced in interpersonal relationships. He did not have any of the classic symptoms of inattentiveness, forgetfulness, hyperactivity, and so forth. In addition, his history showed that he was attentive in school and obtained good grades without conduct problems. His job changes were not caused by lack of focus and/or boredom but because of interpersonal problems.

Q. Aren't boys supposed to be boys? Isn't misbehaving part of learning to grow up?
A. Yes, boys are supposed to be boys and it is generally true that they are more aggressive than girls are. It is also true that younger chil-

dren have more difficulty controlling themselves. The process of socialization starts before school and continues through young adulthood. Youngsters learn to gain more control and self-discipline as they grow older. Children seldom communicate their feelings directly. Misbehaving is one way in which children communicate to others that they are having trouble. Many children misbehave; not all of them are ADDers. Continuous inappropriate behavior is definitely a signal that a child is trying to communicate a problem.

Q. If this is so, then what is ADD and why list the above behaviors as a syndrome that needs professional attention?

A. There is a difference between misbehaving because one is young or immature, or has less control as a younger child, and attention deficit disorder behavior.

Each age group has varying abilities to contain themselves, assert control over their feelings and behavior, and make practical decisions. All of these abilities improve with age, experience, and practice. This process of mastery begins very young and continues as children grow. Normal children make these gains with ease and, for the most part, learn from their mistakes by making better decisions.

Most children with ADD have great difficulty gaining control over themselves, in spite of the positive efforts they make. They need professional attention. A professional can help the parents to work more effectively with their children and help them organize their child's day so the child is more motivated and unlikely to give up. A professional can also assist in providing structure, guidance, and support for parents with their emotional enmeshment.

Q. I am still confused as to why all children cannot make the same gains. Aren't underachieving children just lazy?

A. In some cases, yes. However, there is a distinct population of children and adults that are not lazy yet cannot self-correct their behavior so that they can go forward and get things done. Scientists estimate that approximately 3 percent to as much as 6 or 7 percent of the population falls into this category.

People with ADD have nervous systems that are a little different from their non-ADD peers. Scientists are not clear exactly why, but a few hypotheses have been put forth to explain the ADD brain and how it functions. Many experts believe that the ADD brain underproduces a chemical known as dopamine. When dopamine is in short supply the person feels more agitated, is more easily distracted, experiences less inner quiet, and, in general, has less impulse control. Brain scans have shown that the amount of dopamine in the front part of the brain of ADDers is less than that of their non-ADD peers. Today, it is generally understood that there are distinct biochemical differences in the nervous systems of these two populations. These differences tend to manifest as follows:

- *Inattention:* The ADD child tries to pay attention but he gets distracted and literally forgets that he is trying to pay attention.
- *Impulsivity:* Children who are impulsive sometimes know they are impulsive. They try to contain themselves but cannot because the minute a thought comes into their heads they almost automatically react to it.
- *Hyperactivity:* Children who are hyperactive try to slow down but their nervous system keeps them jittery, fidgety, and revved up nonetheless. Even when they "turn the key" to shut off the engine, it keeps racing a mile a minute.
- *Hypersensitivity:* Children who are hypersensitive, and who become aware of it, try not to let things bother them so much, but a small slight that might seem like a minor irritation for most people hurts them deeply. A severely hypersensitive child may be constantly churning inside, certain the whole world dislikes him or her.

Q. Can different schools or different teachers help my child?

A. The answer is a qualified yes. Schools are set up to educate the majority of the population and that means they are geared toward working with kids who are at least fairly compliant. Children who do not match up to these standards, and this certainly includes most ADD children, frequently have difficulty in a normal classroom. The following illustration might be helpful:

John is kindergarten age. He was diagnosed with ADD and had some problems with anxiety. He attended kindergarten for a few days and his teacher reported to his mother that he was uncooperative, would not follow instructions, and was belligerent. She also said that John was a bad influence on the other children. When she gave the children a drawing assignment, John refused to do it. The more she threatened him, the more belligerent he became. She wanted John out of her class.

John was showing classic signs of being overwhelmed. Both children with ADD and those with anxiety disorders become overwhelmed easily and lose the ability to think clearly, even when it would seem to their obvious advantage. When this happens, they freeze. I talked with John and discovered that he was not sure how to proceed with the assignment the teacher gave him and was fearful of doing it wrong. In feeling overwhelmed, he simply closed down. The teacher misinterpreted his closing down as obstinacy, and further badgered him, escalating his confusion and then his "obstinacy." Because John's teacher could not control him, he got a bad rap.

At his parent's request, John was transferred to a different kindergarten teacher, with whom I spoke. She was able to encourage him, provide more instruction, and soothe his fears. John progressed well and experienced no further problems.

Many ADD children need closer supervision and function better in smaller classes with a structured learning environment. Changing teachers can be helpful if the change includes the kind of teaching relationship he or she needs. The child with ADD needs to be working with a person who understands ADD kids and what they require to learn and interact in a way that will allow them to experience themselves in a positive light. Also, parents need to learn how to interact with their ADD child in ways that will help the child learn how to handle the special challenges facing him or her.

Children with ADD are also eligible, under a disabilities act, to have an individualized educational program developed to meet their needs. (Much more is said about this in future chapters.)

REJECTED PARENTS

One of the most painful experiences for parents is to feel that their children reject them. Children do become angry with their parents, no doubt about that! Sometimes grown children continue to blame their parents for their feelings of low self-esteem and for their troubles in life. This type of emotional blaming hurts the grown child and the parents. The grown child is hurt because blaming prevents him or her from focusing on the issues he or she needs to confront and grow through. Focusing on the past does not change the present or future. Blaming hurts the parents because it is unfair to them as well. In most cases, parents do the best they can. Even if they are hampered by life's traumas, such as divorce, job loss, illness, and so forth, they still care about their children. Their ability to help their ADD children, particularly without some professional guidance, is often greatly reduced when they are experiencing rejection. Many valiantly try to help but find their efforts turned against them as previously discussed.

My own parents were very concerned about me. They did everything they could think of to help me. I was a tough child. My parents worked hard for my siblings and me. My mother went to work in the 1950s to help earn money for the family at a time when women were expected to stay at home. I knew my parents loved me. Yet, as an ADD child, I was unable to experience and accept their love. As you will soon read, my feelings about myself were far removed from what my parents felt about me. My parents were good, concerned, hard-working people. They did the best they could with the resources and knowledge they had.

A sentence from Chapter 1 bears repeating here. I understand very clearly now that the parents' perception of giving love is not necessarily adequate for the child to feel loved.

A PRESCRIPTION FROM THE HORSE'S MOUTH

Looking back on my own childhood, I sometimes ask myself what would have been helpful to me. The first thing that comes to mind is that I would have found some comfort in knowing that I was different from other children but this did not mean something was wrong with me. The very next thing that comes to mind is that I would have greatly appreciated being understood even if it meant others would take a little more time and exercise a little more patience with me. It would have been great to know there was someone who would stick by me as I grappled with this mystery!

If someone had taken me aside, perhaps my mother or a kind teacher, and told me that I was okay, and that all of us were a little different from each other, I would have felt much better about myself. I would have felt better about myself if I had been able to see that many people have to work harder in school and there were programs to make studying easier for me and the many others like me. I would have liked being told that I was smart, that grades had little relationship to intelligence, and that I had special qualities many other children did not have. Each and every one of these points could have kindled my hope and motivated me to approach the challenge of being me in a more constructive way. I believe I would have felt much better about myself and this positive self-image would have definitely encouraged me to keep moving ahead.

If learning tasks had been given to me with the structure and support that allowed me to accomplish my work, I could have more easily esteemed myself, and felt good about being Don.

If we had more conversations and fewer rules, more conversations and less one-way communication, (which I often perceived as "scolding"), my fledgling self-esteem would have found more fertile soil into which I could have sent my roots.

In actuality, it would not have taken much for me to be more relaxed and comforted in childhood. That awareness is, without a doubt, a powerful motivating factor in all my work with parents struggling with ADD kids, and it is my central goal in writing this book. What greater reward could there be than to see that others might benefit from the knowledge gained from one's own struggles?

Chapter 4

Your Child *Can* Change:
Teaching Your Child New Behavior

*Our life is at all times and before anything else the conscious-
ness of what we can do.*

Jose Ortega y Gassith
The Revolt of the Masses

In Chapter 2, I reviewed some of the lessons I learned as a parent.
One of the most significant was that character building needs to be
learned at home. Parents have a unique opportunity to help their children feel good about themselves and develop positive self-concepts.
Furthermore, the ADD child's behavioral tendencies often work
against the very acceptance of their basic needs within the family system. This makes the work more challenging and more necessary.
Building ADD children's solid sense of self allows them to accept
their strengths and limitations and to eventually lead happy, produc-
tive, and responsible lives.

DEVELOPING A PLAN FOR YOUR CHILD

Your child needs to know what to expect from you. Children with
ADD tend to lack organizational abilities, and they have only minimal abilities to consider the consequences of their actions. But there
is a way to provide your child with a sense of order and structure.

Many children tell me they do not know what to expect when they do something "wrong." Sometimes they are punished; sometimes their behavior is overlooked. Other times they are unaware of having done anything "wrong" and they get screamed at, not knowing what "set off" Mom or Dad.

Dustin, a young high school boy, told me that he preferred to talk to his father and avoid his mother most of the time. He said he knew what to expect from Dad. When he was in trouble, he clearly knew he was in trouble with his father. Mom, on the other hand, nagged and lectured him. This confused him, increased his anxiety, and made him feel bad about himself.

James, a fourteen-year-old boy whose parents are divorced, alternately lived in San Francisco with one or the other parent. His father's house was chaotic. There was much screaming and yelling in the home and his father and stepmother frequently fought over how to manage his misbehavior. He was smart enough to play one parent against the other. However, over a period of time, their inconsistent responses to his actions, ranging from physical abuse to overlooking his behavior, became too chaotic for him. He finally chose to stay in his mother's household where his mother and stepfather were in agreement on matters of discipline. It is interesting to note that when presented with a real choice, he chose that situation where clarity and structure were provided rather than the situation where he was manipulating the adults.

I remember when I was young my father liked to wrestle with my brother and me. My ADD energy would kick in and I would soon be out of control. At about sixty pounds I would be intensely trying to pin my father to the ground, not letting up. Out of the blue he would suddenly hit me, striking me with a hard blow. I would get up crying and run to my mother, who then would blame my father for starting the roughhousing. His answer was, "Donny got carried away."

All children need a sense of order, whether or not they have ADD. The ability to organize reality in a way that reduces anxiety is important to all children. The more inconsistent or chaotic the household, the more anxious the ADD children become and the more difficult it is for them to begin developing the skills they so badly need for managing their ADD patterns. So you can see how important it is to provide your ADD child with a sense of structure and safety in the home.

PLANNING HELPS THE PARENT

As the parent of an ADD child, you need a plan as well. A good plan will give you confidence for working with your child and should allow you to meet unexpected surprises with appropriate action. Most parents I meet are bewildered. A good road map can guide you through the vicissitudes of daily life with a challenging child.

Miles, ten years old, lived with his eight-year-old sister and his parents. When I first met him, he was out of control. His parents, both of whom were understanding and kind, had tried everything they could think of to help Miles with his behavior to no avail. As we started to work together, Miles showed some improvement but progress was slow and relapses frequent. Both his parents were reluctant to apply certain disciplines because they were too tired, or they felt that Miles would fuss so much it would only make matters much worse. The *time out,* which consisted of having Miles sit down for a few minutes whenever he got out of control or misbehaved, was part of the road map we had drawn up to deal with specific misbehaviors. After about three months, Miles' father finally agreed to try this tactic. Approximately one month later, he reported to me that this procedure made a significant difference in Miles' behavior. On a follow-up visit about six months later, the father reported that when he consistently applied the time-out chair Miles' behavior definitely improved.

Most adults would not think of starting a business, building a house, saving for retirement, or shopping for a Thanksgiving dinner without a plan. Interacting with an ADD child without a plan might be analogous to driving across the country without a road map in hand. In fact, some people would compare it to starting a trip across the country in a car before even learning how to drive!

Developing a plan is nothing more than having a set of rules that provide structure for you to apply in various situations. A plan will reduce family chaos, give you a sense of confidence, and allow your child to know what to expect from you.

FIVE BASIC RULES

1. Work as a team with your partner.
2. Interact immediately when your child misbehaves.
3. Interact in a consistent manner with your child.

4. Interact in a fair manner with your child.
5. Interact with your child, using positive reinforcement for acceptable behavior.

Work As a Team with Your Partner

As you begin to introduce new learning or behavior it is critical that both parents be in agreement. In most cases, your child will resist change. He or she will test your willingness to implement the new learning. Much of the time the child's old reactions and reflexes will tend to support or reinforce your own habits. Children are very aware and very clever. If there is a hint that both of you do not support the new teaching with conviction, the child will test you and try to play one of you against the other. Be on the lookout for this and, if there are differences in your parenting styles, discuss that issue with your partner out of the child's earshot. Even if you do not immediately feel it, do try to present parental agreement to your child.

Occasionally, you and your partner may have different viewpoints about solving a problem. This is to be expected. It is important to discuss such differences and share your ideas. If, after you have shared your differing opinions and listened to each other, you still disagree, then you must compromise on a common solution. Let one shared goal guide you toward compromise: that you both recognize how important it is to support each other and present a united front to your child. Who is "right" and who is "wrong" may be far less important where your ADD child is concerned than presenting a "unified front."

Interact Immediately When Your Child Misbehaves

From the discussion above, it should be clear when the child misbehaves he or she needs to be confronted immediately. This allows the child to review the inappropriate behavior while it is fresh in his or her mind, think about it, and respond to immediate consequences. If a child teases a sibling, refuses to study, is disrespectful, will not do chores, or will not go to bed on time and is not immediately confronted, a talk by his or her parent later on will have little impact on changing bad behavior. ADD children learn from this that they can get away with irresponsible behavior when they want to and then face a talk sometime in the future. Since the talk usually goes in one ear and out the other, it is seldom of any consequence to them one way or another except that it takes up their time.

If the child is becoming active, is starting to rev up and lose control, the sooner you intervene the easier it will be for the child to calm down. Immediately intervene, directly addressing the problem: "You are starting to get carried away splashing water, Tom. Stop splashing now." This allows the child the opportunity to contain behavior before completely going over the edge.

If the child is already carried away, screaming at a sibling, hitting someone, running wild, etc., a clear and immediate intervention can allow him or her to become aware of poor behavior. Once the child has learned some skills for dealing with his or her ADD behavior, he or she can begin to calm down.

Remember that ADD children are usually not aware that they are hyper or acting impulsively. An immediate intervention is the best way to bring their activities to their conscious awareness. Change will not happen immediately, but stay with your plan and you will eventually reap the benefits. Remember, these are not instant cures, but tenacity and persistence over time will bring the results you seek.

Interact in a Consistent Manner with Your Child

It is important that your interventions be consistent. This means that you need to interact each time the same misbehavior occurs. If consequences are not applied in each case, the child learns that sometimes misbehavior goes unnoticed. If allowed to misbehave sometimes, the child will then develop the habit of trying to see how much bad behavior is allowable. Each time misbehavior goes unpunished, you are actually encouraging the old pattern. This will make your efforts to change, as well as your child's efforts, frustrating and discouraging to say the least. When ADD children are aware of their behavior and know that they will consistently receive positive reinforcement for acceptable behavior and negative consequences for what is not acceptable, new learning begins to take place.

Interact in a Fair Manner with Your Child

This is one of the biggest problems I encounter in my work with families. Some parents tend to either overlook or ignore behavior that is inappropriate. Other parents overcorrect and are too severe in their punishment: small transgressions result in the loss of television privileges for a week or grounding for a month. Frequently, parents will ignore the same misbehavior in the morning that they will harshly punish a few hours later.

When interventions are too harsh the child senses the unfairness and becomes angry. This anger can be manifested in many ways, such as through more misbehavior. In this case, the ADD child's reaction is often one of feeling that regardless of what he or she does, punishment is forthcoming, so why do anything to try to be good? Sometimes the child feels a sense of hopelessness because he or she is unable to change the severe punishment and simply gives up. Often the child is punished unfairly because the parents do not know what is fair; being frustrated or angry, they hold back their anger until they finally explode at the child.

A few years ago, I worked with a family that was having difficulty with their teenage son. He was required to return home immediately after school. He was not allowed to have any friends visit nor was he allowed time for being with friends after school. Phone privileges were suspended. He was not allowed to watch television. He had absolutely no freedom; every privilege had been rescinded. His parents told me that they could think of no more punishments, yet their son would not change. I had to restrain myself from choking the parents in anger. After containing myself, I asked the young man if he saw any reason why he should make any effort to change. He said it would not make any difference. I told him I completely agreed with him, then we opened the session up to discuss how this problem could be corrected.

Nothing can be accomplished by releasing your anger on your child. There is only one goal for applying the types of interventions I discuss in this book: that is, to help the child recognize and choose more effective and rewarding behaviors.

Fair reinforcement is an intervention that is sufficient to help the child choose a better option. Fair negative reinforcement is the minimal intervention that will produce the change desired or help the child choose more wisely.

I cannot emphasize enough that this is one of the more troublesome problems parents encounter: ignoring misbehavior or overreacting and punishing unfairly. In the next chapter I will discuss in particular how to apply fair interventions.

Interact with Your Child, Using Positive Reinforcement for Acceptable Behavior

This is perhaps the most important rule of behavior modification. Children change more quickly when positive reinforcement is applied. Although there are different points of view, most researchers agree that a positive ratio of 4:1 is required to effect a lasting change in behavior. In other words, four positive reinforcements would ideally balance every negative intervention.

When dealing with ADD children, most parents issue many negative commands and comments: "Don't do that! Stop tormenting your sister! Your homework is terrible!" Most families use somewhere between a 5:1 and 20:1 ratio of *negative* intervention to *positive* reinforcement! And, of course, we know what is ultimately achieved in that case: lowered self-esteem, higher anxiety levels, and increasingly negative patterns of behavior.

As parents, you may tend to think negatively about your ADD child. You may be ready to pounce on him or her. That is only natural since they greatly challenge everyone around them. Believe me, I realize that positively reinforcing an ADD child on a 4:1 basis can seem like a superhuman endeavor. But be patient: in the following chapters, you will be learning ways to do this with far less effort than you might imagine.

Chapter 5

Charting the Course to a New Life: Motivating Your Child to Change His or Her Behavior

You know most people live ninety percent in the past, seven percent in the present, and that leaves them only three percent for the future. Old Satchel Page said the wisest thing about this I ever heard.

John Steinbeck
The Winter of Our Discontent

A FEW COMMENTS

The specific techniques presented in this chapter will be very helpful to you in changing your child's behavior and the way you interact with him or her. One of the most important chapters in the book, it teaches you new ways to help your child to both change behavior and improve his or her self-esteem.

You might ask why I did not use these techniques with Manuela when she was young. The answer is: I would have loved to, but I did not know about them at the time. Believe me, learning the skills described here have not been easy for me. In particular, it often meant facing the things I did in the past that exacerbated our problems rather than improving them. During the time Manuela was growing up, I was unaware of the fact that she had ADD or, for that matter, that I had ADD. Even as an adult, my own childhood experiences left me feeling inadequate in many ways. I have no doubt that I worked hard to be successful in the business I was in at the time in part to overcome some of my own ADD traits. My efforts paid off in terms of financial rewards but did nothing to help me understand the ADD experience that Manuela and I had in common. Furthermore, because I had gained a sense of self-esteem by pushing and driving hard and by being a stern taskmaster with myself, I thought these measures would also work for Manuela. I thought that if I just pushed her hard enough she would eventually see things my way. It was not until many years later when she was an adult that I discovered both of us had ADD.

I did not realize that her childhood vision of the world was very different from my own adult vision. In the same respect, it never occurred to me that my parents' vision of life had been very different from mine. Until I started treatment for my own ADD I had never examined the thought that each of us experiences life differently. I was too busy battling my own demons and trying to outrun them.

It has taken me years of work, study, and introspection to realize that I needed to understand Manuela's world and her ADD behavior. By entering her world, I could have set up incentives that were realistic for her, that would have encouraged and motivated her to make better decisions on her own. I could have set up tasks that she could accomplish and, in the process, allow her to experience herself as a competent person. Unfortunately, these realizations did not come about for me until many years after her patterns were set, and I was able to reflect back on my life and my limiting thoughts about myself as well as her. As I worked hard to change my thinking patterns and beliefs, I was actually preparing myself to help others in ways I could not help Manuela when she was growing up. This may be small compensation for Manuela, but our fondest hope would be that others might benefit from our early errors.

ANOTHER LOOK AT ADD

As a child I had trouble doing various tasks that were expected of me. I knew that I was supposed to do something but for some reason could not get going. The best way that I can explain the feeling is that the task was across the room, and, even though I knew I was supposed to do it, I could not move to where I was supposed to be. It sounds like I was simply lazy, but it was more than that. It was as though a thick concentration of air was between the behavior I desired and me. This made it almost impossible for me to push through to the desired end. When I work with children and share with them this type of information, they frequently get excited and realize that I have an idea of what they experience.

Anyone who has experienced a depressive episode is somewhat familiar with this behavior. The depressed person simply does not have the volition, the physical energy, or stamina to execute certain activities. It is a bit different with ADDers. They may have physical stamina but are unable to summon the wherewithal to get things done. Have you ever had the experience of being faced with a task that is just too demanding? It costs too much, requires too many people, takes too much thought? ADD children experience this often, even for something as mundane and simple as carrying out the garbage or doing homework.

Mental and emotional energy can be reduced or blocked just as physical energy can. If you watch a two-year-old child bouncing around the house full of energy, playing with abandon, you wonder where that storehouse of energy comes from. A few minutes later, if the child's mother leaves the house or a new baby-sitter emerges that the child is uncomfortable with, the child's energy suddenly collapses like a balloon when the air is released. Where did the life force go? The answer is that the child's energy has just reconfigured itself in a new manner, going inward rather than outward.

Many people believe that the ADD child is obstinate. In some cases this is true; however, it is frequently more than that. It might be more accurate to say that the child's energy is blocked or not readily accessible. The child does not quite have the wherewithal to get tasks accomplished.

The concept behind developing a motivational system is to help the child develop the needed energy to learn new positive and self-affirming behaviors.

In the previous chapter, we discussed five basic rules. They were:

1. Work as a team with your partner.
2. Interact immediately when your child misbehaves.

3. Interact in a consistent manner with your child.
4. Interact in a fair manner with your child.
5. Interact with your child, using positive reinforcement for acceptable behavior.

In addition to these rules, we will be applying effective methods to
boost your child's motivation. ADD children can make progress in
high-interest activities. By focusing on one desired behavior change
at a time and developing your child's strong interest in mastering that
activity, your child will slowly begin to change his or her behavior.
You will learn to apply effective interventions as your child displays
both positive and negative behaviors.

Many professionals are not in agreement about rewarding a child
for work that the child should be able to do. They argue that the child
needs to learn to be responsible and contribute to the family and his
environment in a meaningful and helpful way. Although this may be
true, virtually all professionals who work with ADD children agree
that this is not the case with attention deficit children. Their ability to
follow directions and complete tasks is limited, as I indicate throughout this book. They do not easily grasp the inherent reward mature
adults find through responsible participation in a family or community.

It has been my personal as well as clinical experience that I need to
stack the deck in the child's favor, so to speak. Stacking the deck in
the child's favor is nothing more than encouraging or enticing the
child to make a different choice from the one he or she is prone to
make. When I speak of motivation, I am including all methods of
encouragement that can help produce the desired behavior, new
learning, or a better sense of self-esteem.

I have listed below a few reasons why it is important to develop
motivational skills to help your ADD child:

- The inattentive child needs special interactions and strong
  encouragement so that he or she can learn to pay attention and
  focus.
- The impulsive child's thought becomes an automatic reaction.
  The child's ability to contain behavior is not as strong as the
  expulsion of desire and energy that gets released when he or
  she moves into action.

The impulsive and hyperactive child lives in the present. The future—later this evening or tomorrow—is too far away to hold this child's attention. The world exists only in the here and now.

The ADD child's nervous system is different from that of his or her peers. The child needs to make a special effort and needs extra motivation to curtail automatic reactions, impulses, negative behaviors, etc.

Learning new behavior is not easy for any of us, but it is particularly difficult for children with a fast nervous system. In a sense, all of your child's current behaviors have been learned in the past. What has been learned can be unlearned, and new behavior can supplant old. This is a task that requires planning and effort on your part as well as cooperation by the child. Encouraging the ADD child to try hard to change unacceptable behavior is a significant part of teaching new learning. The types of reinforcement listed below work best in motivating your child to learn new behavior:

- Verbal encouragement
- Nonverbal encouragement
- Indirect verbal encouragement
- Tangible rewards and privileges
- Point charts
- Negative reinforcement

VERBAL ENCOURAGEMENT

Simply stated, verbal reinforcement is nothing more than praising your child for good behavior. The statements you make that allow your child to feel a sense of self-control and power tend to reinforce or encourage your child to repeat the new behavior because he or she benefits from doing so. The types of praise you can use are virtually endless. I have listed a few that I frequently use:

- "That's right. Good for you!"
- "Nice job."
- "That's really nice."
- "Keep up the good work."
- "Good choice."

- "That's showing good restraint."
- "You've got it now."
- "Nice work, that really helps me."
- "I can see you made a major effort, congratulations."
- "Good self-control."
- "I like the way you cleaned the table . . . sat in your chair . . . cleaned up your room . . . came into the house when I called . . . stopped what you were doing . . . studied when you were supposed to . . . got dressed in time for school," etc.

Verbal encouragement can be any praise you give your child. But be specific to each situation. Focus on actions and avoid general or nonspecific praising such as, "You were a good boy today." Notice how specific the following statement of praise is: "You made good choices today when you stopped teasing your sister each time I reminded you." "You showed a lot of self-control today." "You did all your chores when they were supposed to be done."

Be creative in your positive verbal reinforcement. What spontaneously comes to mind at the moment is probably very appropriate.

NONVERBAL ENCOURAGEMENT

Nonverbal reinforcement is also a good way to encourage and reward your child. Gestures, smiles, thumbs up, a nod of the head, a pat on the shoulder, and other gestures convey praise without using words. Combining verbal and nonverbal reinforcement works well, too. A combination of positive praise and a hug or pat on the back can make your child feel good and helps establish a bond between the two of you that he or she will value.

INDIRECT VERBAL ENCOURAGEMENT

Indirect reinforcement also works well. Complimenting the behavior of your child to your parents, spouse, relatives, or friends when your child is within earshot is another way of communicating praise indirectly. Speaking in the kitchen about your child's good day so he or she can hear it from the living room is another form of reinforcement. You can use this method with your spouse when he or she returns from work or shopping. Speaking on the telephone so the child can hear it is another variation on this theme. If possible, talk specifically about the behavior change so the child will have direct feedback on the behaviors involved. For example, "George, I was so proud of Mike today. He took out the garbage for me immediately after I asked. And he did a really good job on his homework."

I like this type of communication because ADD children probably already hear more than they care to about what a problem they are. Chances are they have been the butt of a number of complaints and criticisms parents have voiced to others. Speaking about them in a positive manner allows them to begin to feel better about themselves and to see themselves in a very different light. Sometimes it can be more effective to hear indirect praise than direct praise. Think about it for a minute. Would you like it if you overheard your boss saying a number of positive things about you to a colleague? Would you feel good? Research has shown that we are most deeply affected when we are praised in the presence of other people.

By combining different types of praise you are able to give your child a lot of positive reinforcement for the same behavior. Remember how important it is to build your ratio of positive to negative reinforcement. Use your creativity to look for new and more effective ways to deliver positive strokes.

TANGIBLE REWARDS AND PRIVILEGES

Frequently, the use of positive praise alone will not be enough to get a child started along a path toward constructive behavior. More powerful reinforcement is usually needed. Tangible rewards and privileges are stronger motivational tools that encourage your child to make the extra effort.

Tangibles are simple rewards you give your child, such as going out for a special treat to acknowledge and reinforce good behavior. Simple rewards allow your child to experience more of what he or she wants or desires through the choices he makes. A short list of rewards might look something like this:

- Playing outside longer
- Watching an extra hour of television
- Staying up later at night
- Having a friend over for dinner
- Going out to have pizza or to a favorite fast-food restaurant
- More computer or video game time
- Renting a movie
- Having a parent read a favorite story

Such privileges can provide extra motivation to encourage your child to exercise more self-control. You might tell your child that if he or she does not argue or fight with siblings all day then he or she will get to pick a video to rent or have a friend stay overnight.

Be sure you do not use these special privileges as threats such as, "You're not going out tonight if you don't stop fighting." Some parents easily slip into this way of thinking. Be alert and remember that you are trying to introduce positive strokes to motivate your ADD child. Later in this chapter I discuss ways to interact with your child if he or she fails to respond to positive incentives.

These rewards can be used as midweek reinforcement for obtaining a certain number of points on the point charts suggested below. Remember the rule: *Children change behavior through positive encouragement, not negative.*

POINT CHARTS

Point programs reward the child for displaying desirable behaviors. Points can then be redeemed for privileges, access to things the child enjoys, or money.

Programs such as this are very effective because points can be delivered immediately. In addition, the parent has the opportunity to reinforce the child's self-esteem when awarding points by adding praise or other positive comments.

The short list above barely scratches the surface of the types of rewards the child can earn. By exchanging points for special privileges, the child can vary his or her rewards and stay motivated to earn more points.

Another advantage of point programs is that the child gets to participate in his or her behavior modification program; the child becomes an architect in drawing up plans for his or her own change.

Point charts can be very simple. Today many children have some computer skills and I ask them to create a point chart on the computer with parental help, if needed. Usually the child delights in doing this.

Children usually have a long list of special privileges they would like to enjoy. Allowing the child to brainstorm with you about such things as bonus awards and the number of points to be exchanged for privileges can be fun for them as well.

Many children like to have money so they can purchase things on their own. Frequently this is a powerful motivator. The points program allows points to be redeemed for money, privileges, or any combination to which you and the child agree.

Sometimes I like to add bonuses. An example of this might be if the child obtains a score above 90 percent in a given week, bonus points or a special privilege is earned (see Figure 5.1). I find that this frequently can be an extra incentive motivating the child to work hard. Other times you can surprise the child by adding extra points to the score at the end of the week when he or she does not expect it. You might say, "I thought you did your chores especially well," or "There were a couple of times during the week that I wanted to compliment you when you were doing good stuff but I forgot to tell you."

FIGURE 5.1. Point Program

CHORES	MON	TUE	WED	THU	FRI	SAT	MAX. POINTS
Feed Dog	X	X	X	X	X	X	6
Clean Table	X	X	X	X	X	X	6
Empty Trash			X				1
Clean Bedroom and Put Toys in Room	X	X	X	X	X	X	6
Water Flowers	X	X	X	X	X	X	6
POSSIBLE SCORE	4	4	5	4	4	4	25
MY SCORE	4	4	5	4	4	4	25

All chores are to be completed by dinnertime.
Mom agrees to remind me twice and give me a choice.
I get a bonus if my score stays above 22.
If I get angry or talk back I will lose a point.

It has been my experience as a therapist that point programs are the most efficient method of behavior change. They have many advantages over other types of reinforcement and incorporate the use of a wide variety of reinforcers. Additionally, they make it easy for the parent to reinforce immediately and effectively, encouraging the strong use of positive verbal and nonverbal reinforcement.

Frequently, it is important to break the day into segments. Sometimes it can be very difficult for a child to avoid the old habit throughout the day. If the old behavior occurred frequently, it will be too difficult for the child to turn in a perfect day to get a token. If the token is too hard to obtain, the child will lose motivation; you have to be flexible and observant, adjusting point earnings on the basis of the child's realistic capacities so he or she can experience the positive reinforcements that are very important to receive.

I try to use a combination of common sense and intuition to determine how the day will be divided. If, for example, the child teases his younger sibling throughout the day, I might make a chart divided into morning, afternoon, and evening sections. Avoiding the old behavior during a specific time period then allows the child to accumulate points.

Remember that children enjoy participating in creating the chart and making decisions on how it will be scored. Younger children who do not have computer skills like to copy suggested outlines of point charts. By doing this they feel they are cooperating with the parents and have a voice in changing things.

Figure 5.2 is an illustration of a typical point program chart. I particularly like it because it clearly spells out the agreements between the child and his or her parents on the chart itself. Upon agreement, the child and his parent could put a star, a happy face, or perhaps a red check mark on each day the duty was accomplished.

Zack

Zack is an eleven-year-old boy with ADD. When Zack came to my office he expected I would join with his parents and blame him for his shortcomings. Following my evaluation, which included discussing the problems this ADD family faced, we decided to work on the problem Zack had in completing his chores. I asked Zack to share his thoughts and feelings about doing chores at home. He was a little reluctant to speak at first, but began to open up as he realized I was

FIGURE 5.2. Typical Point Program Chart

CHORES	MON	TUE	WED	THU	FRI	SAT	SUN
Make Lunch							
Open Blinds							
Clear and Set Table							
Empty Dishwasher							
Wed. Empty Cans	No	No		No	No	No	No
Sat. Clean Room	No	No	No	No	No		No
*Extra Credit Feed Animals Help with Yard							
Total Points	4	4	5	4	4	5	4
Points Done							
Bonus Points							
Percentage							

very interested in what he had to say. He complained that he was tired by the time he came home after school, that he did not like to do chores, he hated the nagging, and so forth.

I told Zack that I thought we could reduce or eliminate the nagging about chores and, in addition, could probably develop a reward system for his work around the house. I told him I thought chores were important and that we could set up a system similar to one he might encounter at a later age when he finished his schooling and began work.

In Zack's case, his parents gave him money for the movies and other activities and, at times, withheld it if they were having more trouble than usual. Zack and his parents agreed on how much he could earn in a week if he did his chores. With this agreement in place we were ready to set up a chore point chart to both remind and motivate Zack to carry out his duties (see Figure 5.2).

As we talked, Zack became very interested in my proposal and participated in determining the chores that would be involved. He made compromises, accepting some chores he did like and getting his parents to trade certain chores he did not like.

We then placed a dollar value on the points he could accumulate. His parents agreed that reminders would be delivered to him twice in a normal tone of voice. Then, if he still had not done the chore, they would ask him what choice he wanted to make. If he chose to do the chore he would get his point. If he did not, he would forfeit his point and, therefore, might fail to get enough points to obtain his weekly reward. I usually start a point chart in this manner. If the child does not respond to the incentive I will have the child lose a point for making a bad choice. I always try to encourage the child to change his behavior through positive reinforcement. In Zack's case, to sweeten the pot we also set an incentive of earning an extra dollar if he scored above 90 percent each week.

I asked Zack to go home and draw up a chart reflecting our agreements and bring it back the following week. Next week Zack brought me the chart illustrated in Figure 5.3.

The results were almost immediate. Zack did his chores and his parents stopped nagging. The new agreement lasted several months, after which I saw Zack and his family less frequently.

On a regular monthly checkup at a later date, both Zack and his parents were back in the Big Struggle. As I questioned Zack, I discovered that his Little League team had won their division and were now practicing on a daily basis. This made it difficult for Zack to do his chores as had been previously agreed upon. We agreed to some adjustments during his intensive practice season and made sure this was agreeable to all family members. On our subsequent visit, Zack and his family had returned to the harmony they had previously achieved.

FIGURE 5.3. Zack's Point Program

ZACKMAN'S CHORES	MON	TUE	WED	THU	FRI	SAT	SUN
Make Bed							
Make Lunch							
Open Blinds							
Set and Clear Table							
Wed. Empty Cans	No	No	No	No	No	No	No
Sat. Clean Room	No	No	No	No	No	No	
*Extra Credit Feed Animals Help with Yard							
Total Points	4	4	5	4	4	5	4
Points Done							
Bonus Points							
Percentage							

Jeshe

Jeshe is an eight-year-old girl who was already diagnosed with ADD when she and her mother came to my office. I completed an evaluation to help understand the problems they faced. One of the problems that troubled Jeshe's mother most was Jeshe's poor hygiene. Jeshe did not like to brush her teeth, comb her hair, wash her hands, or attend to most personal care necessities.

As with Zack, I asked Jeshe why she did not like to take care of her personal hygiene. She said it was not important to her; besides, she was tired and she thought she did it a lot of the time anyway. I asked her what happened when she did not obey her mother on this issue. She replied that her mother would constantly nag and sometimes get angry and raise her voice. I asked Jeshe how she felt when this happened. She replied, "My mom hates me."

I like to ask this question frequently because I know that children think their parents do not like them. I also know that ADD children want to be loved, yet many have a hard time believing that they are accepted and loved because of the disagreements and fighting that takes place between them and their parents.

I asked Jeshe, "If I can get your mom to nag you less and praise you more for attending to your personal needs, would you give it a try?" She said she would. I also told her that it would probably be difficult for her to change this old habit because it was so strong. She agreed that it would probably be difficult. I then asked her what kind of reward or privilege would help her to learn the new habit for becoming more grown up. We talked about a few rewards and she thought that earning some money for behaving like a big girl would help her break the old habit. Earning money seemed like a very grown-up thing to do and she was eager to try.

On subsequent visits she scored around 75 to 80 percent on her hygiene attempts. Her point program is shown in Figure 5.4. This was a definite improvement, but not as good as I hoped we could achieve. She liked not being nagged and said her mother stuck to her end of the bargain. I asked her when she was given the choice between earning money by changing her habits or choosing not to change, why did she sometimes chose not to change? She said that at times the money did not mean that much to her.

I reasoned that two factors were working against Jeshe. One was that she had to wait too long to collect her reward; the other was that

FIGURE 5.4. Jeshe's Point Program

	MON	TUE	WED	THU	FRI	SAT	SUN
Brush Teeth		☆☆	☆☆	☆	☆		
Brush Hair		☆☆	☆☆	☆☆	☆☆		
Wash Hands and Nails		☆☆	☆☆		☆☆		
Get Dressed		☆☆	☆☆	☆☆	☆☆	☆☆	☆☆
Bathe		☆☆		☆☆			☆☆
Brush Teeth = 1 = 2x Day x 7 = 14 Brush Hair = 1 = 2x Day x 7 = 14 Wash Hands and Nails = 1 = 2x Day x 7 = 14 Get Dressed = 2 = 1x Day x 7 = 14							

she was not motivated enough to change. Her mother told me that in the previous week, Jeshe wanted a particular music tape and when her mother offered that as an incentive, Jeshe did better. We decided to find rewards that offered more incentive. As we substituted other rewards, Jeshe was more successful. Jeshe is typical of many younger children who are not sure of what they want. When working with children, it is important to have a list of possible rewards they can choose from to motivate them appropriately.

Raghu

Raghu, a nine-year-old boy, fought constantly with his younger sister. He would tease and scare her while his mother yelled at him. After being reprimanded a number of times, he would become uncomfortable with the coldness he experienced from his mother and would then apologize. After a period of feeling close to his mother he would start up a new cycle of antagonizing his younger sister. When his mother brought the children to me she was in tears and clearly worn out.

Raghu was very sensitive to change in his environment and had trouble adapting to any transition. Unfortunately for Raghu, his grandparents would visit from long distances and stay for long periods of time. During these times, Raghu's acting out would intensify, as this was his way of releasing the tension he felt because of the disruptions these visits required.

Raghu was very cooperative in therapy and participated actively from the start. I tried to find out what triggered his agitation. After several meetings, we were able to identify the things that most frequently caused his misbehavior. Because his teasing was almost constant, I needed to break it down into manageable segments. He gave me a list of the reasons he believed he did not get along with his sister. His list included situations such as fighting over television, Raghu going into his sister's room, and who was right or wrong during an argument.

Next, I needed to break the day into smaller segments so that Raghu could earn a reward for controlling himself for short periods of time.

I also knew Raghu was a very sensitive child and that when his mother yelled at him he would contain his discomfort for a period of time before becoming scared that she no longer liked him. In Raghu's particular case, I felt if his mother could give him reminders in a calm tone of voice and offer him a choice, she would be giving him an opportunity to make a decision that would yield positive results.

It turned out that Raghu was a budding banker: he liked money. We set up a token system that would allow him to earn a little money for each time period. The point program chart shown in Figure 5.5 was set up so that as Raghu tried to change his behavior we could see where it was easier, as well as more difficult, for him to contain himself.

With the information I had learned so far I felt it was time to create our point chart. I set up the usual rules of reminders, choice, and calmness. Then I asked Raghu to make up a chart, with his mother's help, and bring it to me for our next session.

The following week a major improvement had taken place. In that first five-day period, Raghu was able to control his behavior and earn points each and every day.

The next week his point chart showed a dramatic change for the better. Although a very fast behavior change is not unheard of, it is somewhat unusual. I suspect Raghu's mother may have overlooked some minor teasing.

Most of the time, I find that the point chart yields good, but not perfect, results. It usually has to be modified. I tell parents that the point chart is a general template I use to generate new behavior patterns. I require my clients to return the week after we draw up a point chart to customize it to the reality of the child's experiences the previous week.

FIGURE 5.5. Let's Get Along

DATE/TIME	REASONS NOT TO GET ALONG				
	Television	Right/Wrong	Personal Space	Stuff	Tokens
Saturday 9:00 - 12:00					1
1:00 - 6:00					1
7:00 - 11:00					1
Sunday 9:00 - 12:00					1
1:00 - 6:00					1
7:00 - 11:00					1
Monday 9:00 - 12:00					1
1:00 - 6:00					1
7:00 - 11:00					1
Tuesday 9:00 - 12:00					1
1:00 - 6:00					1
7:00 - 11:00					1
Wednesday 9:00 - 12:00					1
1:00 - 6:00					1
7:00 - 11:00					1
Thursday 9:00 - 12:00					1
1:00 - 6:00					1
7:00 - 11:00					1
Friday 9:00 - 12:00					1
1:00 - 6:00					1
7:00 - 11:00					1
Total Tokens Earned					21

This was the case with Jeshe, who was not motivated by the rewards we selected the first week and so we tried new rewards that proved more successful in helping her develop better hygiene habits.

The Value of Points

The success of your program will be partly determined by how effectively you motivate your child to learn new behaviors. Therefore, you will have to spend some time in discussion with your child about the value of immediate rewards (points accumulated in a few days or less), intermediate rewards (points accumulated over a period of one week), and long term rewards (accumulated over a period of a month or so).

It is important to determine how much value each point has. Each point can be converted into a monetary value as well as a redemption value. Many children do not have any idea how much things cost. It is important to help them determine redemption value. Using Raghu's point chart as an example (see Figure 5.5), we agreed one point equals $.20. The maximum he could earn would be $.20 times 21 points, which equals $4.20. A bonus might be worth an extra $1.00. The maximum money that could be earned per week would then be $5.20.

Points could be worth more or less than the monetary value in redemption. Some examples might be:

Short-Term Rewards (One- or Two-Day Accumulation of Points)

Three points   =   Get to choose a video to rent
Six points   =   A friend stays for dinner
                 I get to watch an extra television show
                 I stay up twenty minutes later tonight
                 Mom reads me a bedtime story for fifteen minutes

Intermediate Rewards (Points Accumulated During a Week)

Twenty points = Pee wee golf
                 I get to skip one chore for seven days
                 I get to go to the movies and take a friend
                 I get to have a friend sleep over
                 I get a small toy or game

If a child saves for an intermediate term reward, he or she will not be able to earn daily rewards as well; the points have already been spent.

Long-Term Rewards

Large rewards are special treats that are more costly in time or money than intermediate treats or rewards. Since long-term rewards are achieved over a period of a month or longer, you can choose to be creative. The reward might be a new "hot" video game or the chance to go to a theme park. Pick at least four or five long-term rewards your child would like.

You can also be flexible in how long-term rewards are given. You might want to have your child accumulate seventy-five or eighty points in the chart system like Raghu's and redeem them for a specific long-term reward. As a method of additional encouragement you can also simply reward your child with the special reward if he or she has already redeemed short-term points.

You want to make it easy for your child to earn points quickly, as this will keep motivation high. This is especially true for younger children who have short attention spans.

You can also make up a grab bag for nine, twelve, twenty, or any number of points in which values worth that number of points are in the bag and the child draws out one special privilege from the grab bag.

As mentioned earlier, it is important to have your child participate. You can also help him or her by asking questions such as, "If you had one wish, what would it be?" or "What are things you like to do with your father?" or "What would you like to save money for?" These types of questions help the child to think of rewards that he or she really values.

By now you should have a good idea about putting together a point chart and developing a system of rewards. Throughout the book we will be utilizing these concepts. The token economy will become one of your most effective tools in helping your child to learn new behavior.

As your child learns the new behavior you can gradually phase out the point chart. It is important that you remain liberal about giving verbal reinforcement and occasionally giving surprise rewards. You may want to set up a general chart without specific duties so that you can reward good effort during chores or for displaying a cheerful attitude while helping out around the house.

This then frees you to set up a reward system to get new learning started. It is important for children to help out around the house by doing chores. I believe that daily chores are a method by which children can earn money or privileges and, in the process, experience themselves as attentive to the needs of the environment while making a contribution that others need and appreciate. More will be said about phasing out point charts later in this chapter.

There will be times when positive reinforcement is not enough to effect behavior change. The appropriate use of negative reinforcement combined with positive reinforcement becomes necessary.

NEGATIVE INCENTIVES

I prefer using natural consequences whenever possible. Natural consequences, such as those listed in the next section, can be very effective motivators. It is important to determine ahead of time what natural consequences will follow for specific types of misbehavior. For example, ADD children need to be alerted ahead of time so that they know the consequences of their decisions. The next chapter on empowering your child discusses how to make him or her aware of the choices available.

Loss of Privileges

Natural consequences must be incorporated into your point chart if it becomes evident that positive reinforcement is not producing adequate change. Usually, effective application of the combination of positive reinforcement through a point program and negative reinforcement through removal of privileges will provide the child with incentive to change old behavior. Some examples of negative consequences follow.

- Going to bed early
- Losing television or computer game time
- Sending friends home early
- Removing toys or playthings children are fighting over
- Getting up earlier in the morning if children are late for school

As with privileges that a child earns, there are many ways in which negative reinforcement can be applied. If the child splashes water in the pool, time out of the water can be a natural consequence. If the child starts homework late, television and evening privileges can be adjusted. If the child leaves toys in the living room, removal of those toys as playthings for a period of time can be used.

There will be many instances when it will not be easy to apply natural consequences to help your child change his behavior. In those instances, another type of negative reinforcement will be necessary.

Time Out

Time out is very effective for helping your child learn new behaviors when positive reinforcement does not produce change. Time out should be performed in the following manner:

1. Review the situation. Is the misbehavior one that you have discussed with the child? Is there an agreement that the child will go to time out if he or she does not stop the activity? If so, use the following procedures.
2. Quickly review your personal state. Are you calm? Can you mirror calmness?
3. Approach the child and make close contact so that his or her attention is focused on you (if at all possible).
4. Give the child two reminders that he or she is misbehaving and a choice to stop the activity or go to a time-out chair.
5. If the child continues to misbehave, either guide or direct the child to a prearranged chair.
6. If the child resists, bring the child firmly to the chair. Do not squeeze his or her arms or shoulders. If necessary, hold a piece of clothing (his or her pants) and guide the child.
7. If the child makes promises to quit, begins to argue, promises not to do it again, simply say, "You made a poor choice; now you have to go to time out." If the child keeps arguing, repeat one more time that he or she made a poor choice.
8. *Once the child is seated in the chair, his time does not start until he becomes quiet, stops arguing, or stops trying to get away.* The first few times you do this you may find it necessary to stand next to the chair while the child tries to get up. Just repeat that time out does not start until he or she is able to sit in the chair without making noises and fighting with you.

9. It is important that you remain calm. Do not get caught answering the child or responding to his or her attempts at conversation. Be sure that you are in control! This means you must not get excited, raise your voice, or yell at the child.
10. Many parents have told me that initially it took them up to twenty minutes to get their child to calm down and accept the time out. Most children get the idea after a few minutes, but you should be prepared for some resistance. In time, the child will learn that he is increasing personal time lost by resisting you and will go to the chair to get the time out over with.
11. I like to have the child sit one minute for each year of age: a five-year-old child would sit for five minutes, a ten-year-old for ten minutes, etc. You can vary this slightly.
12. If the child gets out of the chair before his time out is over, place him back in the chair and start his time again from the beginning.

These rules should cover most of the problems you might encounter. Consistency is very important. Each time the child engages in the behavior that warrants a time out, your consistent application will help him or her to change most quickly.

I have had parents repeatedly tell me that until they accepted the idea of time out and applied it consistently, they did not begin to see good results. Most parents report that within a period of two weeks their children were complying with the time out, sitting still, and learning to make better choices.

PHASING OUT THE REWARD SYSTEM

I like to use the point chart for particularly stubborn and troublesome behaviors. But it is important to work on only one major issue at a time. There are a couple of reasons for this. I do not want to overload the child with too much change at once. Another reason is that the best way to change an old behavior is to use the point chart.

The idea behind the motivational systems that I am using is to create new learning. These are not punishment techniques, and it is important to understand that distinction. The parent needs to learn new ways to approach the child and the child needs to learn new behaviors. But these systems work because the child is actually being guided through a process where he or she begins to be capable of self-control and of doing things that result in higher self-esteem. Once the learning becomes easier, I like to begin to phase out the reward system. As the new behavior becomes integrated, a complete phaseout is in order.

One way to phase out the point chart as new learning takes hold is to require more points be redeemed to receive the same rewards. Gradually, I increase the points required and occasionally like to surprise the child with an unexpected reward. When the new learning is solidly established, the reward system can be dropped and dialogue should take place about changing other behaviors. Another way to phase out the reward is to stop awarding points for one or more of the behaviors on the chart when the child has learned the new behavior.

An analogy might be appropriate here. If you teach your child to ride a two-wheel bike you hold the bicycle and make sure that it has training wheels. The training wheels might be compared to the point chart we have been discussing to introduce a new learning experience. As the child's skills increase, you consider removing the training wheels. This, of course, is analogous to removing the point chart for a particular learned behavior. Even though the training wheels are removed, the child is still unsteady and so you help steady the bike when he or she starts to ride, assist the child in stopping, and so forth. This would be the same as praising the child frequently, giving surprise rewards, or special privileges as he or she continues the new behavior without the point chart. Although the new behavior is learned, the child is still a little wobbly. Just as the training wheels are no longer needed, neither is the point chart, yet it is important to continue to reinforce your child positively. I like to work on one behavior category at a time, therefore I recommend that as your child begins to master one desired behavior, the point chart system can be used for the next behavior pattern on your list.

Jeshe was in a position within a few short months to begin to phase out some hygiene tasks, as they became new habits that she performed without thinking. When this happened there was no longer any reason to reward her for continuing the new automatic behavior. She dressed herself without help and brushed her hair and her teeth on a regular basis. These were three tasks we set up on the point chart to motivate her to take care of herself. She still had trouble taking baths, washing her hands, and cleaning her nails. Her mother and I decided to substitute these three new behaviors for the three tasks she had learned. We used the point chart Jeshe had drawn up and substituted the new behaviors we wanted her to learn. Jeshe continued the "old" new behaviors (dressing and brushing hair and teeth) while she learned the new behaviors (taking baths, washing her hands, and cleaning her nails).

Jeshe learned some new behaviors well but needed to improve her learning in other areas, so it was necessary to keep the point chart. In her case other behaviors that fit the same pattern were added. As you can see, there are many ways to phase out a point chart. It is important to keep this in mind so that you can phase out the point chart wisely.

The possible exception to this is allowing your children to earn money by working around the house. This prepares children to enter the adult world and earn a living. It also fosters a sense of accountability and self-value. In this case, once your child has developed the new behavior of attending to chores, you can simply give the child a weekly allowance without the use of a point chart.

This chapter summarizes the motivation system I use in clinical practice to help ADD children and their parents. Through the use of the motivation system ADD children learn to cooperate with parents in making decisions, receive important help in changing old habits, and begin to reevaluate themselves. As your children begin to change their behaviors, a positive feedback loop emerges in which they feel better about themselves and receive acknowledgment from you, the parent, which supports their new emerging sense of self.

MOVING FORWARD

The next chapter deals specifically with the issue of helping your child feel good about him or her self. He or she has already started to do so as you work with the motivational ideas offered in this chapter. The next chapter deals with building upon the base you have already established. The ideas offered will help you to more firmly build the child's sense of self-worth and personal empowerment. Remember, the issue at hand is building self-esteem, not necessarily getting A's in school; we are far more concerned about developing self-confidence and getting A's in life.

Chapter 6

Changing What Happens Inside: Empowering Your Child

That everyone shall exert himself in that state of life in which he is placed, to practice true humanity toward his fellow man, on that depends the future of mankind.

Albert Schweitzer
Out of My Life and Thought

My experience as a parent taught me that much of the time Manuela felt helpless to perform the way I expected. We were involved in a game of control, which is a typical trap ADD families fall into. At the time, I thought we were trying to hold Manuela to certain standards that were important for her development. I reasoned that eventually she would see the logic of my rationale and be thankful for my guidance. When she was younger I was in control; as she became older the balance of power shifted and she gained the upper hand. We were in a tug-of-war that no one could win.

She lost her struggle for control during the formative years of her life. She lost to a barrage of comparisons, admonishments, expectations, and judgments, all of which I applied liberally, waiting for the day when she would thank me.

There was no opportunity for her to empower herself. She lost what ability she might have had to think about herself in a positive or constructive way. She felt "less than" her peers and siblings. She never learned how to feel good about herself or esteem herself. She lacked the confidence to push forward.

She felt unloved. She was angry with me for making her feel this way and angry that she did not like herself. Her self-destructive behavior started very early. In addition to coping with the challenges of her ADD nervous system, she had to carry this load as well. No matter where she went, there was no escape from what she felt.

I believe it is very important for others to avoid the trap I fell into. Since those difficult years I have worked with many children to help them feel better about themselves. There have been many rewards in this work, seeing other families draw together, and seeing children become increasingly able to live happy, constructive lives where they know they are appreciated and loved.

In the previous chapter, we discussed the need to enter the world of your child to understand how he or she views things so that you can set up incentive plans to help him or her change behavior. We also talked about making a plan that you can follow that has a few rules to provide structure.

The focus of this chapter is empowering your child. The guidelines below can help you build your child's confidence and trust while he or she learns new behavior.

- Understand that your child needs special help; let go of dreams and unrealistic expectations.
- Invite your child into the decision-making process.
- Negotiate with your child.
- Allow your child to make choices.
- Praise liberally.
- Use medication appropriately.
- Do not interact with your child or make decisions when you are emotionally upset.

UNDERSTAND THAT YOUR CHILD
NEEDS SPECIAL HELP

By now you probably understand that your child has special problems with attentiveness, emotional fluctuations, impulsiveness, hyperactivity, and various other ADD traits. Your child needs your help, but where do you begin? One of the most important things you can do is accept your child as he or she is. Accepting your child does not mean that you do not want to teach him or her responsibility. This does not mean that you are willing to accept misbehavior. It simply means that you are willing to accept your child's weaknesses as well as strengths; it means you are willing to work with him or her to build from where he or she is right now, rather than wishing he or she was a different child.

It is very important that your child experiences this sense of acceptance. This is difficult for many adults to communicate. We all have dreams for our children. We want them to live full and rich lives. Frequently, the way we envision them succeeding is by following our well-meaning plans. But if the plan does not fit the child, we need to adapt our own perception to the reality at hand.

This does not mean that ADD children cannot and will not live rich and meaningful lives; it does mean, however, that we need to stop trying to mold them to meet our preconceived expectations.

The following brief case history illustrates how difficult this can be for some of us.

Jimmy

Jimmy was about fifteen years of age when his mother brought him to counseling. He was intellectually gifted. He was also an excellent athlete. He had played eight years of soccer in primary and middle school and was starting on his high school track team. He was also an excellent student receiving an A- average in his first eight years of school.

The problem appeared to be Jimmy's procrastination. He was enrolled in a college prep course at school and his grades began to drop. A's became B's dotted with C's. At the end of his freshman year he did not study adequately for finals and failed a class.

Jimmy was very well behaved and well mannered. His gifted intellect allowed him to get through primary school without making an effort. In high school he was faced with the need to study and plan projects, which were foreign concepts to him. As we got to know one another, a pattern emerged. It appeared that when work piled up, Jimmy would become overwhelmed and frightened. He would simply break down. His mother was extremely disturbed by his lazy I-don't-care attitude. She had hoped that he would receive an appointment to the Naval Academy in Annapolis and was already planning to make the appropriate contacts. In his sophomore year, the same pattern of procrastination emerged in spite of our efforts to help him structure hi courses and workload so that he could manage them. He either failed or dropped out of important classes. He also began to skip school and was frequently tardy.

I referred him to a psychiatrist for medication for ADD. For a while the medication seemed to help, but his mother thought ADD was just an excuse for his laziness. Without her support, combined with his fear that something might be wrong with him, Jimmy stopped taking the medication that made life easier for him. I talked to his mother about letting go of her expectations for her son. She thought he was "going through a phase" and was now entertaining ideas of Jimmy attending a prestigious university instead of the Naval Academy.

As Jimmy did worse in school, his mother slowly dropped her expectations to a point where she talked about him attending a local two-year community college. In the meantime, Jimmy began to hate school in part because he lost confidence in himself and because of the vicious fights that he had about it with his mother.

The fights continued and spilled over into other areas of their lives as Jimmy failed more subjects. By this time his mother had drastically changed her expectations; now she was just hoping that her son might complete high school. Jimmy decided he wanted to finish high school and enter the military service as an enlisted man. His mother did not like this decision, but by now Jimmy was in control; the arguing and bickering continued. Finally, he was not able to make the grades any longer in high school and was transferred to an alternative school that he did not complete.

His mother had watched her expectations for her son drop from expecting he would become a cadet to hoping he might graduate from high school. The arguing and fighting created a deep rift between the two of them. Jimmy's confidence was undermined by his trouble studying and by the constant barrage of criticism he had to deal with.

Sometimes parents have trouble letting go, as Jimmy's mother did. She stopped attending counseling because she had difficulty looking at herself. Although she would say, "I know I'm not a great mother," she had extreme difficulty changing the parts of her behavior that were detrimental to her son's progress. Eventually, she insisted Jimmy visit me alone because she believed it was important for Jimmy to have someone he could talk to that could act as his guide or mentor. She cared very deeply for her son; she simply had trouble releasing her own expectations so that she could help him.

Jimmy turned out to be a fine young man. My therapy consisted of supporting and guiding him and helping him to make better decisions. He also began to take medication and is feeling better about himself. He has a good job and likes his work. He knows he eventually wants to do more with his life, but at eighteen years of age he is satisfied to earn some money and be left alone.

This story highlights how important it is for us to accept our children as they are and find ways to nourish them. As they say in golf, we have to learn to play the ball from where it lies.

INVITE YOUR CHILD INTO THE DECISION-MAKING PROCESS

As discussed in the last chapter, it is important to enlist your child's cooperation in resolving behavioral problems as soon as they are able to. I have seen children as young as four or five years old assist their parents in knowing what would help them improve their behavior. The best way to enlist your child's help is to have a discussion with him or her about the problem. You can point out how difficult the struggle is for both of you. I usually begin by asking the child what ideas he or she may have about changing the old habit. You may find that the child does not trust you or will think that you are going to get stuck in the same cycle of talk and struggle again. This is to be expected. You can then lead with a few suggestions of your own: "I'm trying to find ways not to nag you about fighting with your sister. With your help I want to stop yelling at you." Questions to elicit information or ideas can allow your child to relax a little and feel less defensive. "Do you think if I helped you make a better choice it would be easier for you? Suppose I promise not to tell you more than two times to do your chores and then offered you a choice; how would you feel about that?"

Inviting this kind of cooperation for resolving problem behavior is a way of esteeming your child. If you unilaterally hand down new house rules that the child must obey or be punished, you will undermine your child's ability and confidence to work through challenges, an ability he or she will need for managing life in the future.

NEGOTIATE WITH YOUR CHILD

As you invite your child to help you solve problems, you will need to listen to what he or she has to say. If you are making up a list of chores or deciding what time the child should come in from play, you should be flexible where possible. When discussing rewards and privileges you need to find out what would motivate him or her. The child might want to exchange one chore for another, or ask that a sibling not be allowed in his or her room, or that you allow friends to play in the house. You can suggest various rewards as incentives to change behavior, but let the child choose from a list both of you have drawn up.

When developing a point chart let your child draw up the chart. If he or she is too young, let him or her help you make a chart. Involve the child in every part of the process. Ask, "Do you think if I ask you nicely twice to change your behavior, and you can earn points toward a reward, that you will try to act a different way?"

Do not get caught in a trap of being too rigid: "I will not tolerate any temper tantrums," is too rigid; instead, try, "If you choose to throw a tantrum, I will expect you to go into your room and shut the door until you are finished." In other words, you define alternatives and consequences clearly.

Many parents have not listened to their children for awhile. They may fear being caught in an argument or being badgered or manipulated by a budding young lawyer. Your job as parent is to select the behavior that you wish to change and provide the opportunity for complete discussion and brainstorming. I find that I always learn from the children I counsel. At the end of each session I tell the parents that we have not found a perfect solution, only a working hypothesis. As we continue to meet I learn from parents and children what works and what does not. If parents can take this attitude when working with their children, there need be no recriminations if the first plan does not work. The first plan provides the opportunity to learn from one another as mistakes are made. Keep in mind that there is no single one-size-fits-all sort of plan. Because we are all individuals, what works for one may need some special tailoring for another. As you go along, do so with patience. In the beginning you may go through many trials and failures. Take this as an opportunity to listen to your child again, examine your reactions, and renegotiate or rearrange incentives.

ALLOW YOUR CHILD TO MAKE CHOICES

If you follow the guidelines I suggested earlier you would be alerting your child to his or her old behavior twice and then giving the child a choice. In the previous chapter I discussed both positive and negative incentives as well as use of the time-out chair. Before you execute your new plan be certain your child understands the steps you will be taking. Emphasize that the choice is his or hers—he or she will be making the decision whether to continue the old way or change and try a new way. The child will be deciding whether to try the new behavior and gain rewards or continue the old and forego rewards and privileges. In some instances, he or she will face punishment in the time-out chair.

The child has participated in the development of the plan and will be making the choices. He or she is able to feel empowered to make his or her life better. You will be interacting with the child in a way to help him or her slow down and be able to make better choices. The power is now yours to share and enjoy, rather than be caught up in an endless tug-of-war.

PRAISE LIBERALLY

As your child starts learning the new behavior, praise him or her liberally. At the end of the day congratulate your child on the points he or she has accumulated. When the child receives his or her reward, give praise again. Be creative in the ways you let the child know he or she is learning new habits.

USE MEDICATION APPROPRIATELY

If your doctor has prescribed medication for your child, make sure he or she takes it. The medication will slow down your child's nervous system so that he or she has a chance to learn new behavior, providing the opportunity to experience how it feels to be in more control of his or her own actions. For instance, if you take medication holidays on weekends or during vacations do not try to work the new plan to change behavior. Wait until your child is taking medication again before you restart the new learning program. When well managed, medication becomes a teaching tool. Through the medication the child gets to experience a different world, to feel what it is like to have more self-control, and to feel what it is like to get positive reactions to his or her behavior. In this way, the new behavior and new experiences of his or her world become an internal model. With the model in the child's own mind, he or she can always access it and, in time, learn to modify behavior to adapt to this model. Gradually, the child develops the ability to make use of this model rather than the medication to provide self-control and self-esteem. Or, as the child gets older, he or she can use the medication situationally to handle difficult assignments, meet deadlines, or manage tasks that still remain difficult.

DO NOT INTERACT WITH YOUR CHILD OR MAKE DECISIONS WHEN YOU ARE EMOTIONALLY UPSET

If you are reading this book, chances are that you are worn out by the Big Struggle. You probably have tried everything you could think of to help your child behave better. Now you are reading this book and find that you should be calm and collected when interacting with your child. This may seem like a lot to ask, but there are sound reasons for approaching your child in a calm manner. The next chapter deals with skills and insights to help you, the parent, in this most demanding challenge.

Chapter 7

Lessons for Parents

The softest things in the world overcome the hardest things in the world: To lead them, but not to master them—this is a profound and secret virtue.

Lao-tsu

As parents we need to learn new ways of relating to our children. My story in the first chapter points out that I needed to understand my daughter's disability and then view our interactions through a different lens. I needed to break my mind-set that Manuela was just an obstinate and troublesome child. The story I related about Jimmy in Chapter 6 points out that other parents get caught in the same type of rigid thinking as I did. This chapter deals with our need as parents to relate to our ADD children differently.

Most parents with ADD children ask me what they should do. They recognize that they need to learn new ways of relating to their children. As parents it is easy to become upset when our children act out. We become frustrated, confused, angry, and punitive. We raise our voices and begin to yell, threaten, plead, cajole, and resort to a repertoire of emotional responses. Meanwhile, our child, with a sensitive nervous system, begins to withdraw from us, feeling increasingly alienated and alone. As this scenario plays itself out, the child has little, if any, incentive to change.

The material in this chapter deals with parents controlling their emotions and proceeding in a logical and well-thought-out manner to accomplish their goals and help their child. The six-point checklist that follows will serve to help you as you work with your own child:

1. Self-Check
2. Modeling
3. Contact
4. Awareness
5. Choice (Empowerment)
6. Reinforcement

For most parents living with ADD children, the first reaction they have when their child is acting up is a churning of their own emotions. Often, your own feelings can become the biggest challenge as you prepare to discipline your child or help him or her to change behavior. The following questions to ask yourself at these times can help you gain the composure to be successful under these circumstances:

SELF-CHECK

Where am I? Is this behavior pushing my buttons? Am I upset, angry, confused, and frightened? What is my internal temperature? Am I at 95 percent—close to boiling? Am I at 15 percent—pretty relaxed? Should I count backward from twenty, take a few deep breaths? What do I need to do to reduce my internal temperature? It is important that I be aware of myself if I want to draw my child's awareness to himself so that he has the opportunity to self-correct.

Do I need to remind myself that I am learning new behavior, along with my child? Do I need to remind myself that I have a road map, a plan to follow? Can I allow myself to experiment with this new approach so that I can give it a chance? Do I need to remind myself that this will get easier for me? Do I need to remind myself that I have tried the old way and it has not worked? Do I need to step back and look over my own shoulder in order to get some distance from my emotions?

Where am I now? Can I approach this situation with a bit more perspective? Is my internal emotional temperature dropping now? Can I get my curiosity up so my emotions recede a little?

If you have trouble doing the above, at least you are fully aware that you are close to boiling. You know you have to be a little careful.

You are mindful of your situation even if it has not changed much. This is an improvement over your unawareness of your emotional state in the past.

MODELING

You are your child's greatest teacher. He or she literally uses you as a model. This does not mean that the child acts just like you, but he or she does model behavior after his or her understanding or perceptions of your actions. It can be helpful to think of your child as mirroring something about you. At first it can feel disconcerting to approach life this way, but you'll soon see that it can also provide you with excellent information that you can use to facilitate positive change.

Can I hold myself up as a model of self-control? Can I show calmness and not get excited? Can I show I am not upset with the behavior, yet indicate that it is ill advised? Can I speak in a nonemotional manner to help my child learn to manage his or her feelings and behavior?

If I get excited or nervous, the child will match my energy. I need to stay calm to help the child return to a calm state in which he or she is able to pay attention to me. Even though this may be difficult for me, I cannot expect my child to exhibit self-control if I explode. I understand that my explosion becomes a model for him or her to do the same. If I am having a difficult time controlling my own energy, I can at least understand how difficult it is for my child to show self-control.

I want to approach him or her in a calm manner. I do not have to worry about being led into an argument. I do not have to worry about managing a long explanation. I do not have to figure out what to say if he or she minimizes the incident. I have a formula that I can apply to almost every situation (to be discussed shortly). Should the child become upset or angry, that is okay. I will be able to manage that also (discussion to follow).

After practicing a few times, you will gain experience and find out that you can remain calm, thus providing a model of calmness for your child. Whenever you model calmness, it gives your child a chance to learn new behavior.

CONTACT

I need to get my child's attention. This is important: I want to get very close to him or her. This means that I cannot shout across the room to get his or her attention. It means if the child is in another room, I need to go to where he or she is. I need to make contact in such a way that his or her focus is on me and off the activity that is causing the present problem. The very way in which I make contact with my child may help him or her to slow down, become aware of what he or she is doing. I have a chance to contain his or her excited or revved up energy with my approach. My best chance to do that is to:

- get physically close to the child;
- gain contact by calling his or her name;
- make absolutely sure I have eye contact;
- touch his or her hand, arm, or shoulder if possible. (If the child is extremely upset or agitated, I need to use discretion so that my touch does not agitate him or her.)

Once you have made good contact and the child's focus is on you, you can go to the next step. Your contact alone may allow him or her to stop the disruptive activity.

AWARENESS

Describe your child's behavior while being aware of your tone of voice. Once you have established good contact you can raise his or her awareness: "Tom, you are splashing too much." "Tom, you are getting wild." "Tom, you are exciting everyone by making silly noises." "Tom, you are being too rough with your sister." "Tom, it is time to clean your room, make your bed, put your clothes on, go to bed, take a shower, etc." Make sure that the child understands his or her behavior. And make your description of the behavior brief.

Do not get caught up with your child in a conversation about the behavior; do not enter a discussion. Simply describe the behavior. Once you have described the behavior in a calm manner, wait a short period of time. Allow your child to calm down or to change the behavior. Ten or fifteen seconds (use your discretion) is probably long enough before you describe the behavior again. You are calm, so there is no need to raise your voice or use threatening tones.

When you start to use this approach it is unlikely that your child will stop the old behavior with just one description. The old pattern is strong and it will take time for him or her to grasp the new concepts. Do not be alarmed. You are just making the child aware of what he or she is doing. The child is probably hyper, impulsive, or distractible, so he or she will need time to slow down. This is the reason you create space for him or her to have an opportunity to make a better decision.

Do not describe the behavior more than twice! In the beginning, some parents tell me that they have to yell at their children ten or twenty times to get them to stop. Others tell me that until they raise their voices or threaten punishment, nothing happens. They know their children tune out these messages.

The reason for this tuning out is that children understand non-verbal communication very well. They know they can continue misbehaving until punishment is imminent. They will also respond to one parent more quickly than the other. An acknowledged unwritten contract between each parent and the child exists about the number of warnings you each give and how loud or how angry each parent will get before the child is forced to alter his or her behavior.

By following the steps I have outlined you begin to change that old contract and replace it with a new one. Keep this fact in mind whenever you are tempted to repeat your descriptions of the behavior more than twice.

CHOICE (EMPOWERMENT)

Understand that after making good contact and describing your child's behavior two times, he is in a position to make a choice. I follow a one-two-choice formula. I describe the behavior once and ask the child to stop. He may be wound up, excited; I give him a small amount of time to slow down and become more calm. If he does not, I describe the behavior again and ask him once again to stop. Again, I wait as he moves close to choice point.

If the behavior continues, I then confront the child with another choice. This step is important: it implies that the child has an ability to make a choice. You have, to some degree, interrupted his automatic reaction, and you have given the child the opportunity to master his feelings and behavior.

I like to call this the empowerment phase because you now place the responsibility of change in the child's hands! It is his choice. The child becomes the decision maker. You have delivered the ball into the child's court and it is now his job to control it.

The child makes a choice between discontinuing the described activity and gaining a reward, or continuing the activity and sacrificing the reward. If positive reinforcement does not provide sufficient motivation, the choice may then include negative reinforcement.

REINFORCEMENT

As the child makes a decision regarding this choice, you need to be ready to reinforce it immediately. A delay does not produce a change in behavior. Your child lives in the present. Immediate reinforcement at the point when the child has made a choice allows him to learn new behavior. The child not only chooses whether to change behavior but also chooses the reinforcement that you have previously discussed with him.

Each time the old behavior is enacted, apply the above steps. It is very important that you are consistent in addressing the behavior you want your child to change. Do not ignore it sometimes and address it others.

Throughout the interaction phase you need to be aware of your mental state. What is your emotional temperature? Are you calm?

PUTTING IT ALL TOGETHER

If all this sounds like too much to remember, the following is an illustration to show how it would work in a real-life situation.

Let's say that you want to help your child take responsibility to successfully carry out chores that you have assigned. This might be an issue that is particularly bothersome to you because the child never completes his chores. Perhaps the chores get completed on an irregular basis, or the child does them poorly and you are tired of completing them for him and going through the struggle to motivate the child. You also have agreed that a particular chore is to be started by 4:00 p.m. Let us also say that you have agreed that the reinforcement will be a token to be redeemed for some value at a specific time in the future. You are ready to start your new behavior modification program!

First, you become aware that you need to confront your child because he has not started an agreed-upon chore. You remember your six-point checklist: self-reflection, modeling, contact, awareness, choice, reinforcement. Your approach would go something like this. Realizing that it is 4:00 p.m. and the child has not started to clean the kitchen, you would then ask yourself:

1. What is my internal state? Am I relatively excited or am I calm? (Self-Check)
2. It is important that I model self-control. (Modeling)
3. I want to get very close and obtain his attention. (Contact)
   At this time you go to wherever Tom is and get physically close to him.
4. First Reminder: "Tom, you have not started to clean the kitchen."
5. Wait ten seconds or so. Second reminder: "Tom, you have not started to clean the kitchen yet."
6. Choice: Wait another twenty seconds. "Tom, you are at choice point. If you do not start cleaning now, you will not earn your bonus point."

As you finally get down to describing the consequences, Tom slowly starts to work in the kitchen. You have done a good job at this point. You checked in with yourself. You modeled calmness, and you made good contact. You also did not shout across the room. You are ready to go to the last step, which is reinforcement.

"Tom, you have earned another bonus point!" "I like the way you made a positive choice. I know you probably preferred not to do the chore. Good decision!"

Notice how you have reinforced Tom three times. You gave him a bonus point for his chart and you complimented him twice!

You have covered the main points in our theory chapter. You applied reinforcement effectively. You reinforced your child immediately, you did this consistently, your choice of reinforcement was fair, and you were able to apply positive reinforcement.

Additionally, you did not raise your voice. You did not convey any negative energy. You indicated that his lack of activity was undesirable, but there was no indication that you did not accept him as a person.

Had Tom not started work in the kitchen, he would have chosen poorly. You gave him every opportunity to respond and make a better choice. If he had chosen poorly, you would have said, "Tom, you have now chosen to lose your bonus point." But you still would have remained calm. If Tom repeatedly chose poorly and his behavior did not begin to change, you would simply review your positive reinforcers. Perhaps they would not have been strong enough. You would modify your choice of reinforcement and, if necessary, choose a negative reinforcement.

A lack of change in behavior generally means that you have not provided sufficient motivation to effect new learning. With your understanding of behavior modification you would review your steps and check to see that you followed the basic steps. This being the case you would rethink your reinforcers and try new ones.

Chapter 9, "Putting It All Together," summarizes the most frequent problems parents have when introducing new behavior or new learning. The six-point checklist is a good way to review the methods you used to change your child's behavior.

Chapter 8

New Perspectives on ADD Medication

There is nothing either good or bad,
but thinking makes it so.

Shakespeare
Hamlet

Many parents are still anxious about putting their children on medication. I hope to clear up some of the confusion on this issue. But first, it is important for me to state that I am not a medical doctor. I do not prescribe medication. However, I do work closely with medical doctors in my therapy practice and I would not consider working with ADD children without this kind of professional support.

Over the years, I have clearly seen the benefits of medication for ADD children. In fact, most of the children I work with would make minimal gains, if any, without appropriate medications from a qualified specialist. Clearly, when a solid program of behavioral modification therapy is used in conjunction with medication, many children do extremely well at learning more rewarding behavior. In many instances, as the person grows older the need for medication minimizes and eventually is not needed.

In presenting the material in this chapter, I lean heavily on Phil Kavanaugh, MD, and Bruce Wermuth, MD, my professional colleagues at the clinic.

For many children, if not most, psychostimulants are the first medications doctors use in treating childhood ADD. Why are they prescribed? Children who are hyperactive, impulsive, oversensitive, and inattentive calm down when they use these medications. Psycho-stimulants that normally speed up a non-ADD person's reactions have the opposite effect on ADDers. They cause the brain and nervous system of ADD children to operate more slowly. Non-ADD children have internal "wiring" that inclines them to be more reflective, less impulsive, and less environmentally sensitive. Stimulant medication helps ADD children to be more like their non-ADD peers, slowing down their typically "hair trigger" reactions, and increasing their ability to focus.

Researchers have identified upward of seventy neurotransmitters in the human brain. Of this large number, only a handful of these chemicals appear to directly affect our sense of well-being. The names of some of these chemicals may be familiar to you: dopamine, serotonin, norepinephrine, and PABA. When produced in normal quantities, these natural chemicals contribute to our sense of well-being.

ADD children appear to produce insufficient amounts of dopamine. The addition of stimulants to the child's brain does not directly add dopamine as such; rather, it allows the dopamine that is naturally produced by the child to be used more efficiently, which is important. The stimulant medication increases the release of dopamine and slows down the rapid absorption of this chemical into the child's system so that this normal and natural chemical stays in the brain longer where it can do the work it is intended to do.

The end result of this form of medication is that it strengthens the child's ability to block out irrelevant thoughts and impulses and allows the child to focus. Without medication, the child's thoughts and attention might travel in a million directions. With medication, the child can stay tracked on a single thought more easily. With medication, the child can find and employ a "brake pedal," giving him or her better mastery over impulses and better self-control. As hyperactivity decreases, the child tends to develop a "thicker skin," and is less prone to react to every little thing.

This same medication given to a person with "normal wiring" would actually cause the nervous system to speed up. I believe it is this paradoxical effect that creates so much concern for people.

Some teens and adults with "normal wiring" have abused this medication and given it a bad name. It is relatively inexpensive, is a favorite of the drug culture, and probably will remain so. Even so, there is no denying that, when used along with a good behavior modification program, this medication is safe and very effective in helping ADD children to literally turn their lives around.

Some people are fearful that such a medication might introduce their children to street drugs and lead them into drug abuse. My concern is just the opposite. I have worked with too many teenagers and young people who have dropped out because they had ADD and could not measure up to society's standards. They turn to street drugs in a desperate effort to reduce their pain. This, in my mind, is one of the risks of not using medication wisely and monitoring it appropriately.

I have not yet found a mother whose ADD child was treated with these stimulants who did not swear by that treatment and what it did for her child. Nor have I found a mother who, having experienced the benefits of these medications, would consider discontinuing it without a doctor's advice.

Medical doctors (psychiatrists) prescribe other medications as well. Tricyclic antidepressants such as Elavil or Tofranil are frequently used. Sometimes stimulants and antidepressants are used in combination. A small percentage of children do not respond to stimulants, so other medications are occasionally used.

It is not uncommon to see children experiencing other disorders such as depression and/or anxiety. ADD frequently does not stand alone. A good diagnosis will help you identify these problems and better understand them. In such cases additional medications are frequently used.

It is not my intent to introduce you to the doctor's medicine cabinet. I only hope to increase your understanding of the dopamine enhancers (stimulants) so that you may be more relaxed and confident about helping your child.

Less than 10 percent of the children I work with do not take medication. I find that these children are able to make gains nonetheless. I have learned through experience that the parents' money and my efforts are wasted if children do not take medication when needed. If you want to help your child by using the material I present in this book, I urgently suggest you have him or her evaluated for the possibility that he or she can be helped by medication.

The correct combination of medication and behavioral modification therapy will simply allow your child to maximize his or her ability to begin to take control of problem behavior. Once on this road to more constructive and satisfying behavior, that new existence produces its own positive reinforcement. Children feel better about themselves because they can achieve a level of self-mastery that previously eluded and frustrated them.

In helping our children to master their emotions and behavior, appropriate medication, taken as indicated, is an important first step. However, this is only the first step. Although these children will have somewhat greater control over themselves, new behavior patterns need to be learned and old maladaptive behaviors need to fall away. Stimulants and other medication help to restore the brain's natural chemistry so that the child can successfully listen, process information, make choices, and control behavior. These medications may give your child the capacities to learn the new behaviors, but you must supply the lessons.

Chapter 9

Putting It All Together

Slights and insults are the common lot of humanity, loss and gain.
. . . . The most difficult and the most essential of all perfection is
equanimity, especially for a layman who has to live in an ill-
balanced world with fluctuating fortunes. In times of happiness
and adversity, amidst praise and blame, he is ever balanced.

Narada
The Buddha and His Teachings

A SUMMARY OF THE STEPS

If you suspect that your child has ADD, review the information in the first chapter of this book. Your child could very well be misbehaving because he or she is angry and wants to hurt you. The child could be misbehaving because a major transition has occurred in the family, such as moving to a new school that the child does not like, a death in the family, or perhaps there has been a divorce. When children are unable to manage the stress of change, it is not unusual for them to act out.

Children will act out for other reasons as well. If your child is depressed, has a childhood anxiety disorder, or other mental or emotional problems, it may impair his or her ability to control behavior.

One of the key indicators of ADD is that behavioral or attention problems are usually present by the time the child is six or seven years old. School reports from teachers frequently bring this information to the parents. One of the problems in determining if children have ADD of the inattentive type is that this behavior pattern may be overlooked because many teachers suspect ADD only when they observe hyperactivity. For this reason, too many girls with ADD are overlooked, and names such as spacey and daydreamer are substituted to explain this behavior.

As you review the material in the first chapter you may believe that your child does exhibit ADD behavior. But do remember that this information is not meant to be used for diagnosis. Should you believe your child has ADD, investigate further. Get your child tested for ADD. Child psychiatrists, some pediatricians, some psychologists, some marriage and family counselors, and some clinical social workers can test your child if they are familiar with ADD treatment. Inquire throughout your community until you find a professional who has experience working with this specialty. You may find the school your child attends provides testing of this kind. Contacts with your child's teachers are important. The specialist testing your child most likely will want information from school resources.

Do not assume that just any professional has expertise in this area. Be willing to ask questions to determine whether the person you are talking to has experience with ADD diagnosis and treatment.

Following an evaluation, your child should get a medical checkup by a child psychiatrist or pediatrician knowledgeable in ADD. Chapter 8 gave a summary of why medication helps ADD children.

Some family physicians prescribe medication but do not always refer parents to professionals who help with behavior modification. However, most experts with experience in treating ADD feel that medication alone is not enough. Your child will have to unlearn old habits and learn new ways of behaving. Medication will help make this task easier and help your child to gain better self-control. But it is not the magic bullet. Teaching new behavior is essential.

When interacting with your child to help him or her change you will be most effective when you apply reinforcement as follows:

- Reinforce your child immediately after he or she displays the behavior.
- Apply reinforcement consistently.
- Apply reinforcement that is fair and most effective for the behavior you are treating.
- Use positive reinforcement as much as possible.

These rules arise out of behavior modification theory and first-hand experience working with ADD children. Behavior theory teaches that all behaviors are learned, whether taught consciously or not. The purpose of this work is to create new learning as efficiently as possible. Additionally, the principles of behavior modification theory give you a road map so you may proceed in a simple manner to handle almost any situation you may encounter with your child. Familiarity with these principles will give you an understanding of what you are doing, what works, and why it works. This allows you to be consistent as you carry out your plan to help your child.

APPLYING THE BEHAVIOR TECHNIQUES WE DISCUSSED

Decide on a behavior that you wish to change. If your child does have ADD, you most likely will have a large list. It is important to pick one behavior at a time and work on it. Establish a priority list instead of trying to tackle everything at once.

If the behavior is not complex you should not make up a point chart. A sampling of behaviors you can change without setting up a point chart follows:

- not going to bed on time
- not studying at an arranged time
- leaving the house late for school
- misbehaving in a store
- coming home late
- mealtime problems
- fighting over a toy

As you gain practice working with your child you will get a better idea of behaviors that you can work with directly and those that will require more elaborate planning.

DISCUSSIONS WITH YOUR CHILD

You determine the behavior you wish to change and then discuss this behavior with your child.

1. Let your child know that you will help him change by informing him of the poor behavior and giving him an opportunity to make better choices.
2. Let the child know the sequence you will follow: Awareness—Awareness—Choice.
3. Let the child know what the reinforcement will be—both the positive and negative.
4. Tell the child you agree not to shout or raise your voice, that you are dissatisfied with his behavior, not with him.
5. Tell the child when the new learning program will start (the sooner, the better).
6. Let the child know that he will be making the decisions; the choices will be his to make.

Having completed the above steps, you are now ready to begin. Let us say that your child is refusing to go to bed on time. You are ready to apply the following principles.

SELF-MONITORING, CHOICE, AND REINFORCEMENT FOR THE PARENT

Self-Check

Where am I? If I am upset, I need to calm down. It is very important for me to take charge of my emotions if I expect my child to take care of his or her emotions and behavior.

Modeling

I need to control my behavior. If I get excited or rev up, my child will match my energy. If I approach my child in a calm manner I can actually help him or her to slow down. I definitely do not want to scream, shout, raise my voice, or verbally accuse and/or shame my child.

Contact

I need to move close to my child to get his attention. I need to make contact so that my child's focus is on me and not on the activity. If I do so, my child has a very good chance of breaking his energy. I want to call his name. I want to achieve eye contact. I may want to touch him gently.

Awareness—Awareness—Choice

I will describe the child's behavior clearly, make him aware of it and ask him to stop. If he does not stop I will do the same again after a short interval. If the child does not stop the second time, give a reminder. I will tell my child that he is at choice point and will have to make a decision. I remind the child of the consequences behind his choices.

Reinforcement

In the previous example, I am teaching my child to take responsibility for going to bed on time. Let us say my child makes a good choice. I reward him with the reinforcement I have chosen such as tucking him in bed, complimenting him, or perhaps letting him listen to the radio for fifteen minutes longer.

If he does not respond by going to bed, I then need to apply the negative reinforcement we have decided upon. I might close his door if he likes it open. If he likes to be kissed and tucked in then he loses that amenity. I might have him go to bed fifteen minutes earlier the next night. I may have to vary my reinforcement to find out what is the most effective way to motivate him.

I want to remind myself that old habits are stubborn; sometimes new learning takes a little while. My goal is to improve the irresponsible behavior, not just punish it. I am looking for changes in a positive direction, not overnight success.

USE OF POINT CHARTS

If the behavior you wanted to change were more complex, difficult, or repetitive, you would then want to use a point chart.

Once again, decide on the behavior that you wish to change. Next, discuss this with your child. Then choose the type of chart you want to make. If possible, have your child draw it up. Let him or her pick out stickers or markers that you will use. Determine the maximum number of points that can be accumulated in one week. The value of points could be a dollar figure or they could represent various privileges. Discuss exactly when a token will be earned, if any tokens will be lost, and if time out will be used as a negative reinforcement. I like using a grab bag. In this technique, earning a certain number of points allows the child to reach into a bag and randomly select one of several possible privileges.

Remind your child that you are going to change, too. You agree not to shout or yell at him, but will remind the child in a nice way when behavior needs to be changed. Many children are encouraged by knowing that they are not going to be yelled at. Remind the child also that he will be given two reminders and then a choice.

When I tell children that their parents will not yell at them but will remind them in a nice way that they are doing something inappropriate, they like the idea. I tell them that this is Mom or Dad's part of the bargain.

Learn from your child. By working with behavior modification as I have presented it, you can learn from what works and what does not. Sometimes your child can tell you why he or she was not motivated. Other times you will have to use trial and error until you find something that does work.

Remember that you will be learning new responses and behaviors as you start working with your child. I tell parents this in the first few sessions, as I help patients make up point charts and decide reinforcement measures. Expect to make adjustments, as you learn what works and what does not work with your child.

Some of the more frequent reasons parents have difficulties changing behavior are:

1. The child is not taking medication according to the prescription.
2. Parents do not follow procedure. They yell, nag, etc., and do not live up to their end of the bargain.
3. Parents are not consistent in confronting each instance of misbehavior; some are caught and some are overlooked.
4. Parents choose punishments that are too harsh and the child gives up trying to improve.
5. Parents do not use the time-out chair constructively.

6. Parents get caught discussing, arguing, and fighting with the child instead of following the Awareness—Awareness—Choice formula.

7. Parents are not in agreement about working with the child, so the child is either caught in a battle between the parents or has one parent side with the child, which weakens the authority of the other parent.

8. The child does not like the new changes, chores, etc., and the parent allows this as an excuse.

9. Parents work on too many issues at one time. Overly ambitious parents can overwhelm the child. Work on only one or, at the most, two behaviors at a time to avoid overwhelming your child or causing him or her to feel inadequate.

10. Expect gains but not perfection. Your child has ADD and still will be challenged by his or her nervous system. This entire process is going to be a long lesson in patience for you.

WHAT AGE SHOULD MY CHILD BE TO BENEFIT FROM THE INFORMATION SUMMARIZED?

Children benefit the most from this type of work when they are between ages four and fifteen. By the time your child reaches the middle-teen years he or she is physically much larger and has gained more independence. Many of the techniques, such as the time-out chair, simply will not work. Parents of teenagers need to approach ADD problems in a different way. Part III of this book discusses how to work with teenagers as well as different types of problems you are likely to encounter.

PART II:
SPECIFIC PROBLEM BEHAVIORS
(WORKING WITH CHILDREN
AGES FOUR TO FOURTEEN)

Chapter 10

Taming Aggression

Man must evolve for all human conflict a method which rejects revenge, aggression, and retaliation.

Martin Luther King Jr.
Speech at Civil Rights Movement

Many ADD children have trouble controlling their aggressive impulses. If the child does not learn that aggression is not okay, he or she carries these impulses and behaviors into adulthood where the consequences become increasingly serious.

Unfortunately, most media, including newscasts, glamorize aggression. It is as if society not only condones but also encourages violent behavior. In the wake of this, battered women's shelters filled with beaten women and children abound. The cost to the victims of aggression as well as the aggressor and the society (via police and court costs) are beyond calculation. Yet we continue to glamorize aggressive behavior, basing our subjects for books, movies, and television around it.

If we want to stop this trend and help our children make better choices, we need to do it when they are young. When we do not confront aggression, children learn that aggression is okay. The aggressive child becomes the aggressive adult.

Parents I have known through our work together list a variety of issues that have motivated them to seek help. Performance in school, homework problems, and generally unacceptable conduct get top priority. If the conduct problems include aggression I ask them to work on this behavior before anything else. A few more weeks or months of bad grades concerns me less than failing to curtail aggression *right now.*

When I speak of aggression, I include not only hitting or striking, but also threatening others with harm, pulling, holding, or touching in an aggressive manner, or any behavior that is frightening to another person.

When you decide to confront aggression, I suggest applying steps that we have outlined in previous chapters.

First, evaluate the effectiveness of your child's medication. Is he or she more aggressive just before the next dose is due? Is there a drop-off effect of the medication in the evening? Is the medicine working as well as it did when the child first started taking it? If you believe the child is not getting optimal benefit from the ADD medication, you should check with the child's doctor. The dosage may be too low, too high, or a different kind of medication might be indicated.

Second, discuss the issue of aggressiveness with your child. It is important that you list each and every kind of aggressive behavior that he or she engages in so that the child understands clearly, and exactly, what behavior is to be discontinued.

I suggest making a list of the specific forms of aggression. Include examples of each type of aggressive behavior that you want your child to control. This list of aggressive behaviors will form the basis for your point chart as shown in Figure 10.1.

FIGURE 10.1. Controlling My Aggression

I will stop . . .	Mon	Tue	Wed	Thu	Fri	Sat	Sun
Hitting my sister							
Punching her							
Touching her							
Threatening her							
*							

*If positive reinforcement is successfully used, I can chart reward points. If I need to use the time-out chair, I can still use the chart to monitor progress.

Aggression generally requires negative reinforcement to learn new behavior. Nevertheless, I like to try positive reinforcement first. If positive reinforcement is tried first, then the boxes can contain reward points. The case history of Raghu (Chapter 5) showed that a reward system could work to contain aggressive behavior. It was not necessary for his mother to use the time-out chair.

If you find that positive reinforcement is not enough to motivate a change in behavior, be prepared to apply negative reinforcement. It will be clear to you in a short period of time if your efforts to motivate your child in a positive way are not working. Frequently, combining positive and negative reinforcement can be very effective. In such a situation, the child would be choosing between gaining points and avoiding the time-out chair.

Third, make a point chart. Keep in mind that more than any other behavior, acting out aggressively must be confronted each and every time it occurs.

Fourth, it is very important to provide your child with an appropriate outlet for anger. As you discuss this new behavior program, let the child know that it is okay to be angry but not okay to hurt himself or herself or someone else in the process. Explore ways the child can release his or her feelings appropriately. You might let the child go into the bedroom and scream, or hit a pillow or bed. Give the child a small telephone book to tear or a towel to twist. Sometimes drawing or coloring his or her feelings, or doing other artwork, can be helpful.

Try to be imaginative with your own child. Get his or her ideas. (I worked with one sixteen-year-old boy who hung a punching bag in his room and would work out with it when he became angry.)

Fifth, as the child learns to contain his or her anger, supply plenty of positive reinforcement. Compliment the child on his or her progress.

When intervening with an aggressive child, it is very important to follow the "contact rules" and make certain that you get your composure before you attempt to contact the child. Follow the list, outlined in Chapter 7, that is reviewed in the next section. If your child is aggressive, it may be difficult for you to interact in a calm manner. Be prepared!

PARENT'S COMPOSURE REVIEW

Self-Check

Am I relaxed? What can I do to calm down? Most important, am I angry? How can I contain my anger so that I do not speak aggressively or touch my child in an aggressive manner? I do not want to ask my child to control what I cannot.

Modeling

My child is carried away, out of control. I want to model control. If I get excited and rev up, it will not help him or her. I want to model restraint. It is very important that I do not yell, shout, or use verbal abuse to correct behavior.

Contact

I do not want to yell across the room. I want close physical proximity. That way I have a chance to become the child's focus of attention, and this alone may help him or her to gain self-control. I want to get close, call him or her by name, look the child in the eye, and, if appropriate, touch him or her gently.

Awareness

Now that I am close to my child, I have his attention. I can make the child aware of his actions. This is my reminder stage when I tell the child clearly how he or she is misbehaving and ask the child to stop.

In the case of aggression our Reminder—Reminder—Choice rule is changed. Give only one reminder, wait only a few seconds, and then give your child a choice.

Choice

The choice for the aggressive child is immediate cessation of activity or the time-out chair. Make this very clear.

Reinforcement

You have completed your six-step procedure. Your child will make the decision and you will apply the reinforcement. If time out is the method of negative reinforcement you have chosen in this situation, I repeat the rules of time out here so that they are fresh in your memory.

TIME-OUT REVIEW

- Intervene immediately.
- Send your child to a time-out chair to begin to cool down. For aggressive behavior, I like to increase the length of time in the time-out chair. One-and-one-half to two minutes for each year of age is appropriate in this situation.
- If your child will not stay in the chair, stand behind him and gently hold his shoulders.
- Time begins only when your child becomes quiet. Any outbursts start the time again.
- Do not allow your child to vent any anger at you. It is very important that this is stopped. Should he yell, rage, or become aggressive with you, extend the length of the time out.
- It is very important that you return to a system of positive reinforcement as soon as the incident is over. You might say, "You are getting better control; you only had one time out in two days."

Kyle

Kyle is an eight-year-old boy who was aggressive with his younger sister. He frequently punched, squeezed, or hit her. Other times, he would threaten her with a beating if he was in a bad mood. When Kyle's mother and father came to me for help, they were at a loss as to how to handle Kyle. His mother was worn out and close to giving up.

In the process of getting to know more about Kyle and his family, we decided to refer him for medication. Then Kyle and I talked alone. He told me that he did not like his sister and thought she was a nuisance.

We decided to try positive reinforcement with Kyle first. We made up a point chart to help him. It was clear the following week that no improvement had been made. I discussed the use of a time-out chair and told his parents how to use it effectively. They had reservations about the idea but were willing to try anything.

The following week they reported that Kyle would not sit in the chair and would argue and fight with them when they tried to enforce it. I told them to carry Kyle to the chair, and if necessary, hold him in it and let him know that time did not start until he was quiet. I also told them that it might take up to two weeks for Kyle to begin to contain his behavior so that he would accept the chair peaceably and get the time out over with quickly.

In subsequent weeks, they used the chair in the manner I recommended, and reported some improvement in Kyle's behavior. However, I knew that they were not consistent in using the time-out chair. I reminded them of the importance of consistency when using negative reinforcement.

Finally, after a few months, Kyle's father told me that he was getting it. He reported that he had been applying time out consistently and Kyle's behavior had improved noticeably. He also said he realized that whenever he was lax, Kyle would begin misbehaving again.

Kyle's story demonstrates the importance of persistence in working to curtail aggressive behavior. When his parents first began making serious efforts to change his behavior, they often found themselves too tired or distracted to intervene each and every time Kyle acted out. However, when they did make the effort on a consistent basis, they found that Kyle began to learn to control his aggressive impulses.

PROBLEMS IN DEALING WITH
AGGRESSIVE BEHAVIOR

Your Child Hooks You into a Discussion:
"She Started It"

Aggression is aggression is aggression! There is no excuse and no explanation that justifies it. Do not allow your child to distract you with an argument. Stick to the format: Awareness—Awareness—Choice. Name the aggressive behavior each time, reminding your child that this is unacceptable no matter what the provocation. This may take a little practice, but it works.

Your Spouse Disagrees with Your Approach
or Does Not Support You

Your child's new learning cannot take place until your spouse and you are in agreement. You may have to enter more discussion to work out this issue. Point out that the old way has not worked and suggest that you both give the new method a fair chance. If you still cannot agree, you need to seek outside help before you can start the new learning with your child.

You Are Not Consistent in Confronting Each Aggressive Situation

This is one of the more common reasons children do not change. The child must learn that aggressive behavior is *never* acceptable. There are many reasons for not intervening each time. Sometimes we are too tired. Sometimes we are not convinced that intervention is important or effective. Sometimes we do not catch each occurrence.

My answer is to confront your child's old behavior whenever you are aware of it. That is the best you can do. It should be sufficient to teach new learning. Work cooperatively with your spouse; take turns. If you are too tired, do not be afraid to ask your partner for support. When you first begin this campaign you may simply need to dig deep into your reserves and find the extra energy you need. This can be a real stretch, of course, but the goal is a critical one, and one you cannot treat it lightly.

You May Not Be with Your Child Throughout the Day

If this is the case, then consistently apply the new techniques when you are home. If your spouse, parent, or someone else takes care of your child in your absence, explain the behavior modification steps to them and ask them to follow the procedure.

Your Child Is Too Large to Direct to the Chair or Carry to the Chair

You can generally work with this method of time out until your child is about fourteen years of age. If your child is too large to carry, you may simply accompany him or her to the chair. Time-out rules are the same. If your child is revved up, you can say, "I will wait until you are ready to walk to the chair, but your time does not start until you sit quietly." Do not try to physically force a child who is large enough to resist you in a significant way.

Your Child Is Older Than Fourteen Years of Age

If your child is obedient, you can use this method. If your child has had trouble containing aggression, it is unlikely you can use this method as a way of introducing behavior change.

CONDUCT DISORDER

Children who are neglected, physically abused, or extremely angry sometimes develop what is known as conduct disorder. This is characterized by the tendency of such children to act out against others in ways that reflect the abuse they themselves have suffered. In effect, these youngsters will hit or hurt others because they want them to feel as bad as they do. ADD children are at far greater risk of developing aggressive habits than are their non-ADD counterparts. This is another reason why it is very important to contain aggression when these children are young. The older they are, the more difficult it will be for them to learn new behavior.

Some of the indications that a child or teen has this disorder are as follows:

1. The child bullies, threatens, intimidates others, or initiates physical fights.
2. The child shows cruelty to people or animals.
3. The child has used a weapon, such as a bat, brick, knife, or other dangerous object, to harm others.
4. The child has mugged someone, engaged in extortion, or purse snatching.
5. The child has forced someone into sexual activity.
6. The child has stolen items or broken into someone's house.
7. The child has run away from home.
8. The child has been truant from school before age thirteen.

If your youngster exhibits more than three of these behaviors, you should definitely seek professional help for your child.

This list may appear disconcerting, but it is important for you to have some awareness of conduct disorder so that you can get help for your youngster if he behaves in a way that seriously violates the rights of others.

The ideas discussed within this chapter, when implemented consistently, should be very helpful in managing aggression. If you try these approaches and find that your child still has trouble containing aggression, it is time to seek professional guidance.

Chapter 11

Temper Tantrums

It was a shrill murderous scream, repeated a dozen times with grizzly intensity. It rent the silence to tatters and curdled the blood . . . everyone was too frightened.

Dr. James Lloyd Bowman
Pecos Bill

Many parents literally live in fear of their child's temper tantrums. They dread going into public places with their child, tormented by the thought that he or she might erupt in public. If you have ever known a child who is prone to tantrums, you can certainly empathize with these beleaguered parents. Parents have told me that they leave their child at home and sacrifice their own social activities to avoid such unpredictable public displays.

But what exactly is a temper tantrum? We sometimes think of it as a mysterious force that overpowers the child. The child may even seem "possessed" when in the midst of it. On the other hand, the child's parents feel an array of emotions—confusion, powerlessness, impotence, embarrassment, shame, and sheer anxiety.

A temper tantrum is little more than a display of rage acted out without restraint. A child may throw a tantrum to release extreme frustration; another child may have difficulty maintaining control of his or her temper. Other children have temper tantrums because they know no other way of communicating their emotions. Still others do it to control, frighten, or teach their parents a lesson. In most cases, temper tantrums become a means of controlling others. Be assured that temper tantrums are not a mysterious force; the child is not possessed. Children can be taught to control their tempers.

As with aggressive behavior, it is very important to put a stop to temper tantrums. They represent a serious form of misbehavior that should be dealt with before other types of misbehavior are corrected. As with aggression, when we do not confront and stop temper tantrums they are frequently carried into adulthood. When temper tantrums are not stopped, there is an assumption on the part of the child that losing control works.

When losing control is coupled with aggression, the child learns that he or she can terrorize the household. When adults manifest this type of behavior, consequences can be very serious. Although some child and adult battering is the result of conscious, intentional physical abuse, more of it results from the batterer's loss of self-control.

WHY DO CHILDREN THROW TEMPER TANTRUMS?

One of the reasons children throw temper tantrums is that their parents model this behavior to them. Some parents engage in tantrums with their partners, finding that they can only get their way when they threaten or use these kinds of tactics. I have worked with some families where one or both parents lose their tempers and throw tantrums. In instances where both parents engage in this behavior, the child is constantly modeling inappropriate behavior; in such cases, it is unreasonable for the parents to expect their child to change. Where only one partner engages in this type of behavior and the other partner is deeply concerned, it is less of a problem to help the child gain self-control.

Sometimes children throw temper tantrums because they have learned that this type of behavior gets results. I have talked with many adults who are afraid of their children's tantrums. Some parents abandon the behavior modification process when the child throws a full-blown temper tantrum. Sometimes, if the child has been punished, restricted, disciplined, or grounded, a good temper tantrum might loosen the sanctions, if the parents are intimidated by it. Other times a child might want to get attention and believes the only way to do so is to throw a temper tantrum.

Other parents are chemical substance abusers and lose the ability to control themselves. The image of the drunken parent arriving home while the rest of the family hides from his or her rage is far too familiar to many people.

The bottom line is that the child experiences some type of gain in losing his or her temper. The child usually attempts to control others to get his or her way or release anger, or both.

DISTINGUISHING BETWEEN TEMPER TANTRUMS AND DISRESPECT

Everyone would probably agree that lying on the floor kicking and screaming, shouting or yelling at the top of one's lungs, and loss of control in this manner falls into the category of temper tantrums.

But what is the difference between disrespectful behavior, such as shouting or talking back, and temper tantrums? I believe it is important to make a distinction between the two types of behavior because the way in which you approach your child will be different in each situation.

I believe the difference is one of degree. The difference can be in the intensity and duration of the experience as well as in the purpose. Another difference between tantrums and disrespect is that the child deliberately controls the tantrum. Frequently, tantrums are meant to control the parent to get some type of gain from that behavior. This type of temper tantrum is a full-blown production. It is a prolonged period of high-energy release that has a significantly longer duration and amplitude than its cousin, disrespect.

Disrespectful behavior, on the other hand, usually is not controlling behavior. The child does not act disrespectful in order to get his or her way. In fact, the opposite frequently occurs. A parent will usually be hesitant to give a child something if the child is being mean or nasty.

Disrespectful behavior is usually a result of impulsiveness, thoughtlessness, and the need to release small amounts of anger immediately. The behavior is enacted and quickly dropped. It is seldom prolonged after the words are out of the child's mouth. Much of the time it is an automatic response.

STOPPING TEMPER TANTRUMS

There are different ways of stopping temper tantrums. I suggest using one of these three methods: ignore the tantrum, remove yourself, or isolate the child.

Ignore the Tantrum

Some parents find that they can ignore the tantrum. If the temper tantrum is used to control the parents in one way or another, or to "punish" the parent, the child is rewarded when the parent gives in, gets upset, or remarks in any way about the misbehavior.

When the "reward" is removed, the motivation to continue the tantrum is also removed. As the tantrum is consistently ignored, the child learns that there is no gain in this behavior.

The key word is consistency. This means that if the child lies on the floor screaming, the parent pays absolutely no attention and continues his or her activity. The parent acts as if the child is not present; this means that the parent does not look at the child or give any indication that the child is engaging in any misbehavior.

In order to use this procedure the parents need to check in with themselves and determine whether they can completely ignore all such behavior on a consistent basis. Many parents overestimate their ability to do this. If you believe that you can ignore tantrums on a consistent basis, I suggest you try this method first.

Remove Yourself

With this procedure you simply leave the room. The moment a tantrum starts you say, "I refuse to listen to this," and then immediately leave the room. Make no other comment at all. When the tantrum is over, wait about five minutes and return. If your child threw a tantrum when you asked him to do something, ask or tell the child to do the same thing as if nothing had happened. If another tantrum starts, leave the room and repeat the same procedure.

The first time you try this you will probably find that you have to repeat the procedure. It may take your child many trials to learn new behavior.

Never get into a discussion or an argument about leaving the scene of the tantrum. As with the previous methods we have used, give your child no explanations.

This procedure sounds simple; nevertheless, some parents find it difficult to execute. As mentioned previously, check in with yourself and your partner and determine whether you can carry out these procedures.

When this method is carried out correctly and consistently, you will find that new learning generally takes place quickly once the child understands that there is no reward in having a tantrum.

Another advantage of using this method is that if your child holds a temper tantrum outside in the backyard or at the park you can simply walk away from him or her and apply the same procedure. Simply tell the child once that this behavior is not acceptable inside or outside the house.

If you try this method, and for some reason find that you cannot do it, or if you do not get positive results in a short period of time (within two weeks), follow the next procedure.

Isolate the Child

This method is similar to the use of the time-out chair as discussed in Chapter 5. The major difference is that there is no choice or reminder given to the child.

First decide on a room in which you will isolate your child. The room should have few, if any, distractions to entertain the child. A laundry room is excellent. If you do not have a laundry room, another room with little to distract the child will do. Use the child's own bedroom as a last choice.

The instant your child starts a tantrum tell the child to go to the room. If the child will not go willingly, lead the child to the room. If the child is large enough to physically resist, guide him or her to the room.

As with the time-out chair, the amount of time the child is kept in the room is a minimum five minutes after he or she regains self-control. I generally like to add an additional minute for each year of age. If the child tries to leave the room, you will have to monitor the door just as you needed to monitor the time-out chair.

It is very important to remain calm. Do not get caught in answering the child or responding to the tantrum. Simply let the child know that this type of behavior is not tolerated in your house. When the child leaves the room, do not talk about the tantrum or discuss it in any way. If your child had a tantrum because he or she did not want to do what you told him or her to do, tell the child again what you want. Sitting in the isolation room is not a substitute for following directions! If the child has another tantrum, repeat the above procedure.

During the initial stages of this new learning experience your child will be testing you. You should be prepared to immediately and consistently apply this procedure. If this is done, you should begin to obtain good results. Many children learn in a shorter period of time to avoid the unpleasant consequences, while others have more trouble containing their anger. Should your child take a longer time, you need to accept this and allow your child the space to manage anger in his or her own way out of your range of vision.

If you still have a problem with tantrums after following these procedures, it would be wise to check with a therapist who works with behaviorally disturbed children.

Chapter 12

Teaching Respect

There were times when Brer Rabbit pushed folks so far they couldn't help but want to get even with him. . . . By and by, it got so bad they didn't know what to do.

Joel Chandler Harris
More Adventures of Brer Rabbit

Recently, a parent told me that although her son's grades had improved and he was less aggressive, he was still uncooperative and nasty. When asked to help take groceries out of the car, to shut the door, or to help in the smallest way, the boy would answer "No," or "You do it," or just run ahead. The parent was very upset because her son was completely unappreciative of all her efforts to care for and help him. We talked awhile and, as I questioned her further, we decided to work on helping this child learn to have a more respectful relationship with his mother.

I experience this problem quite often. Many children are unappreciative or take their parents for granted. Other children are verbally abrasive or even abusive with their parents. Some children have an inflated sense of entitlement. Other children are "bothered" by their parents and let them know it.

I lump these types of behavior under the category of disrespect. Disrespect can take a great variety of forms. Nevertheless, the multiplicity of forms can be dealt with in the same way. The following steps will help you to teach your child to be respectful.

First, make up a list of all disrespectful behaviors. Be thorough. Take your time. The checklist that I use (see Figure 12.1) can be used

FIGURE 12.1. Checklist of Disrespectful Behaviors

Checklist of Disrespectful Behaviors	# Times Per Week
1. My child talks back to me	
2. My child ignores me when I speak to him	
3. My child interrupts when I am speaking	
4. My child yells at me	
5. My child takes things from me	
6. My child pushes or tries to hit me	
7. My child says "No" to me when I ask for a favor	
8. My child says "Do I have to?" or "Why me?" when I ask for something	
9. My child deliberately does things to annoy me	
10. Other disrespectful ways my child speaks to me	

as a starting point to identify your child's behavior. You will have to individualize it to fit your particular experiences.

When you have completed your list you are ready to determine how frequently your child is disrespectful. Review the past week and make a log of disrespectful behaviors. Use the list in Figure 12.1 as a simple checklist. If you do not trust your recall, start recording incidents this week. If the behavior occurs less than once a day, but at least once a week, score one for that behavior. Record the average number of specific behaviors each day. When you have your daily totals for each behavior, you are ready to make a point chart.

Make a chart with the data you have accumulated. On the left of the chart count the number of times your child engaged in the old behavior each day. At the bottom of this column total the number of times your child was disrespectful during the week. In the boxes under the daily headings, record the number of times your child engages in disrespectful behavior while you are teaching new learning. This chart will give you a way to measure your child's improvement in respectful behavior as he or she learns to gain control over this habit.

Select appropriate reinforcements. The information in Chapter 5 discusses in detail how to work with your child to set up a reward system that is effective.

After you have recorded the particular disrespectful behaviors your child engages in, and have drawn up a chart as in Figure 12.2, you are ready to start your new learning program.

FIGURE 12.2. Respect Chart

RESPECT								
Old Score	**My Behaviors**	**M**	**T**	**W**	**T**	**F**	**S**	**S**
6	I talk back to Mom	2	1	1	1	1	3	0
3	I interrupt Mom	1	0	1	0	1	2	1
2	I yell or shout at Mom	1	1	1	0	0	1	1
5	I ignore Mom's requests	3	2	2	1	2	0	0
16	My improved score	7	4	5	2	4	6	2
112	Week of 7-23-01 Totals	New Score: 30						

Your child will most likely need some coaching to learn respectful behavior. He or she may have no positive models to draw from or few ideas about how to improve the way that he or she talks with you. You may need to prepare yourself so that you will be able to demonstrate better ways for your child to exhibit self-expression. To be prepared, I suggest the following procedure:

1. Review your list of disrespectful behaviors.
2. Write out alternate ways of speaking or behaving. Try to enlist your child's ideas when creating this list.
3. List the disrespectful behavior and the improved way or ways your child could behave or speak.
4. Discuss the alternative behaviors at a time when your child is not misbehaving.
5. Post the list where it is easy for your child to see.

A sample of such a list follows.

IMPROVING MY BEHAVIOR LIST

Old Way
1. I talk back to Mom.
New Way
1a. I ask Mom nicely if I might be able to do what I want later.
1b. I ask Mom nicely if I can do something else I would like to do.

Old Way
  2.   I interrupt Mom.
New Way
  2a.   I wait until she is finished talking on the phone . . . to someone else . . . etc.
  2b.   I ask Mom nicely if I can speak to her briefly.

Old Way
  2.   I yell at Mom.
New Way
  3a.   I do not yell at Mom. Instead, I tell her I am upset, angry, hurt, or however I feel.
  3b.   If I am angry I go to my room and hit a pillow, the bed, or something else safe to hit.

Old Way
  4.   I ignore Mom's requests.
New Way
  4a.   I do what Mom asks.
  4b.   I ask if I can do it later.
  4c.   If I am studying or working, I ask Mom nicely if I could skip it this time.

You are now ready to start changing your child's behavior.

1. Discuss the behavior you wish to change with your child.
2. Let your child know you will help him or her to change by mentioning misbehavior as it occurs and giving him or her a way to behave differently so a better choice can be made.
3. Let your child know what the sequence will be: Reminder, *example,* reminder, choice.
4. Discuss the reinforcement and the respect chart that you will be using. Encourage your child to help you design the behavior chart.
5. Tell the child you agree not to yell or raise your voice. Also, be sure he or she understands that you are dissatisfied with the behavior, not with the child.
6. Let the child know when the new program will start.
7. Let the child know that he or she will be making the decisions and choices.
8. Review the respectful behavior list with your child.

PARENT'S COMPOSURE REVIEW

As you implement the new learning program, be sure you follow the standard procedure for modeling calmness as discussed in Chapter 7, reviewed in brief here:

Self-Check

Where are you emotionally? Are you calm? If not, what can you do to calm down?

Modeling

I want to model calm behavior. I cannot expect my child to do what I cannot do.

Contact

I want close physical proximity. I definitely do not want to yell or shout across the room. My calm approach can help my child to think and slow down. I want to get close, look him or her in the eye, and, if appropriate, touch my child gently.

Awareness

I want to remind my child that his or her behavior is disrespectful. I suggest new ways he or she might behave from the respect behavior list that we have previously discussed.

If the child has not stopped the disrespectful behavior, I want to make him or her aware that he or she is continuing to misbehave.

Choice

At this point, the child either stops the disrespectful behavior immediately or chooses to continue the old behavior.

Reinforcement

I reinforce immediately. If the child chooses respectful behavior, I immediately use positive verbal feedback. I mark the chart as agreed upon. If the old behavior continues, I apply negative reinforcement, if necessary, and award no points.

If your child does not show improvement within several days, you may need to apply the time-out chair to break the old behavior pattern. If you use the time-out chair, your child will be making a choice to gain a reward or select the time-out chair. Review the information on using the time-out chair in Chapter 5 if you need to refresh your knowledge.

Teaching your child to be respectful requires that you be alert to verbal disrespect and bring it to his or her attention immediately. Consistent intervention is very important when working with this particular behavior.

Chapter 13

Time for Chores

And do not say regarding anything, "I am going to do that tomorrow."

Koran
18:23-24

Many ADD children have problems doing chores. Many parents I have worked with have told me that getting their children to do chores is a troublesome task. Their children forget, procrastinate, promise, forget again, become upset, do inadequate work, grumble, talk back, and in general make the parent feel miserable as they lock horns on this issue. As a parent, I know how easy it is to feel it is not worth the effort to go through the struggle of getting your children to do chores. Sometimes it just seems like less work and hassle to do the chores ourselves.

For the ADD child, chores are particularly troublesome. Their tendency to forget is both conscious and unconscious. In addition, they characteristically rush through unpleasant activities, procrastinate, leave tasks incomplete, and get bored. All these make chores difficult for them to accomplish unless they are highly motivated.

It is also easy for us as parents to draw the conclusion that if we can just get the child to study and behave better in school we will put up with problem behaviors in other areas. Why rock the boat?

Looking back on my own experiences as a parent, I know how easy it is when struggling with this issue to sometimes end up acting like a child. That means getting excited, screaming, yelling, threatening, coercing, overlooking, ignoring, overcorrecting, reacting too severely, punishing unfairly, and, in general, losing control. Outside the house, in the community, or on the job we would never allow ourselves to behave in the ways we sometimes do at home. We absolutely know this type of behavior is counterproductive when trying to help children learn new and better ways of doing things. But it can feel extremely frustrating at times and that is when it is easy to slip into these counterproductive behaviors.

I believe children should do chores because it teaches them responsibility and holds them accountable to a certain standard of performance. It also teaches them that life is not a free ride, that they need to learn to cooperate and contribute to the household, just as they later will need to do to hold a job and contribute to their community.

This chapter will discuss how to motivate your child to do chores and avoid those Big Struggles that make us want to throw our hands up in utter despair.

HOW TO MOTIVATE YOUR CHILD TO DO CHORES

Before you start, you want to make sure that your chore list is age appropriate. Most parents have a reasonable idea of chores appropriate to their child's age. However, if you think you could use a little guidance, ask a few parents who have children your child's age what chores their children do.

Make a list of the chores you want your child to do. Review the list with your child. The purpose of reviewing the list is to get your child's feedback and participation. You may find that he or she will want to strike a compromise with you by trading one chore for another. The following list was for Bill, a thirteen-year-old boy.

Regular Chores

1. Feed dog daily (seven days, one point each day)
2. Vacuum and dust twice a week (two days, one point each day)
3. Wash own laundry weekly (one day, two points)
4. Either clear or set the dinner table nightly (six days, one point each day)
5. Clean room on Saturday (one day, three points)

Bonus Chores

1. Help Dad clean the garage on weekends (one day, two points)
2. Help with yard work on weekends (one day, two points)

Compromise Chore

1. Straighten up living room (seven days, one point each day)

As might be expected, Bill did want to trade chores. In this case, he disliked feeding the dog. A compromise was worked out with his mother and a trade of chores was decided upon. She agreed to feed the dog and he took over her job of straightening up the living room daily.

Work with your child to agree upon the number of points that can be earned for each chore. In the previous case the maximum number of points that Bill could earn was $7 + 2 + 2 + 6 + 3 = 20$ points (excluding bonus points).

It was also agreed upon that if he did not get a perfect score Bill could earn extra points by doing bonus chores on the weekend to build his point total. He was allowed to do this as long as he did not fall below 85 percent of points on his regular point list. In his case it meant he had to earn seventeen points or more to qualify for bonus points.

Having determined the number of points that could be earned, you need to assign a value to them. Chapter 5 of this book discusses in detail how to do this.

Notice how Bill's participation was included in every step of this process. A give and take took place, some changes were made, and compromises and allowances for slips were included. Bill liked to earn money, so a monetary value was placed on the points he earned. If he earned a perfect score he also earned a bonus. Bill participated in determining the value of points. This family worked together as a team and, as a result, everyone was pleased with the new agreement.

Figure 13.1 was the point chart Bill's family used.

Review the information in Chapter 5 if you need to refresh your knowledge of point charts. Once the point chart is drawn up, you are ready to proceed with the new learning experience.

FIGURE 13.1. Bill's Point Chart for Chores

Chores	Points	Max. Pts.	M	T	W	T	F	S	S	Total
Feed Dog	1	7								
Laundry	2	2								
Table	1	6								
Vacuum	1	2								
My Room	3	3								

Maximum Points = 20

Bonus Points (Yard or Garage) = 2

Subtotal _____

Bonus Points _____

Total Pts./Week _____

I have found that children really dislike being told what to do several times. But that presents a problem because, as any parent knows, most children need to be told several times before they do what is asked of them. In many households, the reminders turn into nagging, yelling, or some other type of behavior that the children tune out. Children actually know at what point in the nagging or yelling the parent really means business; as a result they will not do what they are asked until that point is reached. Oddly enough, many children tell me they do not feel good about the nagging and yelling, yet they do not seem able to make a correlation between the nagging and their own behavior that brings it on.

It is important to make this connection for the child—to promise to stop nagging and yelling. Tell your child that you will ask them two times in a civil and respectful tone of voice. Most children like this. Be sure that you clearly define for your child that the second reminder to do a chore places him or her in a position to make a choice. The child learns that he or she makes the choice to either practice the new learning or forfeit a privilege or reward. Emphasize the fact that the child is the choice maker.

Once you have set up the rules, always check yourself to make sure that you uphold your end of the bargain. Most parents do, and find that they get good results. Even in cases where the results are not as expected, you would feel good about avoiding the struggle and not becoming upset. When this plan does not work as you wanted, review the reward system with your child and find out why the child was not motivated. You might need to try different types of rewards or the removal of rewards. Quite frequently the child participates in reworking the point system or reveals why he or she was not motivated. In my practice, it has been rare when any stronger negative reinforcement other than removing points is necessary.

One of the reasons why this approach works is that ADD children are forgetful. The reminders are made in a way that it becomes harder for the child to forget. Another reason for success is that the ADD child's natural tendency to procrastinate is reduced because procrastination past a certain point means loss of a privilege. In addition, the child's motivation to do the work is heightened by a well-thought-out incentive program. Most ADD children function well in a structured environment. This system provides structure and consistency so that your child will know exactly what to expect. Most children like positive strokes, and find that they are easier to obtain when their parents are helping them work with their ADD tendencies.

Having completed your point chart you are ready to introduce the new learning. Imagine it is time for your child to complete the first chore. Being true to old habits, he or she procrastinates, argues, forgets, etc. You are now ready to follow the outline we discussed earlier in which you check in with yourself to make sure you are going to model correct behavior and then communicate your message appropriately to your child (Chapter 7). A summary of this procedure follows.

Self-Check

Where am I? Am I upset that my child is not doing his or her chore after all the work and time I have spent on this issue? I need to be careful not to show that I am frustrated or upset. I do not want to model behavior that is counterproductive.

Modeling

I need to control my communication. If I get revved up the child will get excited, too. I need to approach him or her in a calm manner. Yelling, shouting, or raising my voice is counterproductive.

Contact

I need to move close to the child and get his or her attention. I need to make contact so that the focus is on me, and not on what the child is doing. If I do this, I have a good chance of breaking his or her energy pattern. I want to call my child by name; I want to achieve eye contact; I want to physically touch my child if I feel it is appropriate.

Awareness—Awareness—Choice

I will let the child know that he is ignoring me, talking back, procrastinating, etc., and remind him it is time to do the chore. If he does not do it immediately, I will give him ten or fifteen seconds, then give a reminder again that it is time to do the chore and that he is getting close to choice point. If he does not do it within ten seconds of my second reminder, I will give him a choice to do the chore and gain the reward or to forfeit the reward.

Throughout this procedure I am paying attention to my own trigger points and speaking to my child in a calm manner.

Reinforcement

I reinforce appropriately. If the child chooses the chore, I compliment him on the good choice and mark the point chart as we agreed upon. If he chooses not to do the chore, I tell the child that he failed to earn points that have value to him.

SUPPOSE THIS DOES NOT WORK

The above method of teaching your child to do chores should work most of the time. If no real change occurs after a week of trying this method then you need to find out why. I mentioned earlier in the book that I always learn from the children. When an intervention does not work, I need help from the child to find out why it failed. That, of course, is the responsibility of the adults in a child's life.

I might ask the child why he did not do chores. "Bill, it seems that you were not motivated to do your chores. Can you tell me why?" The most frequent types of problems I encounter with chore schedules are briefly outlined below:

1. The child is not taking his or her medication.
2. The parent does not follow procedure. Dad yells, nags, etc.
3. The parent is not consistent in following up each time the chore should be done.
4. The parent gets upset and punishes the child.

5. The parents do not work together; one is less consistent than the other.

6. The parents get hooked into an argument or discussion about doing the chore instead of simply reminding the child and giving him or her a choice.

7. The parents are trying to do too much and are working on other behavior problems as well as the chore routine.

8. The parents need to rework the reward system with the child because it is not producing the motivation required for change to occur, or they may have to use some negative reinforcement by deducting points.

9. The parents need to listen to the child to hear what he or she has to say that may be helpful. The child can tell you that he or she took on too much, has trouble organizing his or her time, would rather do some chores on another day or at another time. If the child just complains without giving you information, ask him or her questions that will elicit the feedback you need.

EXAMPLES OF TYPICAL PROBLEMS
I HAVE ENCOUNTERED

Zack

Zack, a thirteen-year-old boy, had success when the chore program began but started to have trouble a few months later. In Zack's case, it turned out that he had become active in Little League and his team had won their championship. The coach increased the number of practices, which took time away from Zack's afternoons when he would normally do some chores. The extra practice also caused him to be more fatigued when he finally got home. By the time he ate dinner and studied, he had very little time left in his day. When I met with Zack's parents it was clear that the chore program needed modification during the boy's increased schedule with Little League. Once we did this, Zack and his family got back on track.

Jonah

Jonah, a fourteen-year-old boy, did well as we introduced the chore program. Like many children he eagerly participated in setting it up. We met for a few months and things went smoothly. After that I did not see Jonah for a while. About four months later, I received a call from his parents saying that Jonah was not cooperating at all.

We immediately scheduled a meeting during which I learned that Jonah had made a typical boyish mistake through carelessness and impulsiveness. The details do not matter; the consequence of it was that his parents became angry and grounded him for a long time. It was very clear to me that the punishment far exceeded the crime. Jonah was angry, and told me that after this happened he did not want to work with his parents anymore. Jonah added that as he began to stop doing chores, his mother started yelling at him to do them at which point he would tune her out.

I asked his parents if they would reconsider their decision about punishing Jonah for his transgression. They agreed. I also asked them to follow the procedure of simply reminding Jonah to do his work as we originally agreed upon. After these agreements were made, I told them I wanted to see them in a week. When we met the following week, the chores were getting done and the family was pleased with their progress.

Jonah's problem is typical. Frequently we will agree upon introducing a new behavior, such as doing chores, and the new behavior program starts out smoothly. Down the road, as the child misbehaves, many parents tend to overreact and punish too severely. The child becomes discouraged and gives up on the new program; if he or she is feeling deeply hurt, the child will sometimes revert back to old behaviors.

These stories illustrate that problems do occur. But most families can and do work through such problems when they follow sound guidelines and involve their children in the process. When the chore schedule does not work, it is usually because the suggestions are not being carried out or because parents run into one of the problems outlined above.

By now you are probably realizing that parents can learn to avoid the tug-of-war for control by listening to their children and involving them in the solution process. There needs to be structure for this to occur. The above guidelines should provide you with enough structure to allow this process to continue.

Chapter 14

How to Help Your Child with School

After supper she got out her book and learned me about Moses and the Bullrushes, and I was in a sweat to find out all about him; but by-and-by she let it out that Moses had been dead; so then I didn't care no more about him, because I don't take no stock in dead people.

Mark Twain
Adventures of Huckleberry Finn

Most ADD children experience problems in school that need to be addressed. And as parents it is not easy to ask our child's teachers for special help. Unfortunately, many teachers are not well informed about ADD, which further complicates this problem. Nevertheless, schools are aware of legislation that requires children with a disability to receive appropriate help.

Public Law 94-142 was passed to guarantee equal education for all children. All school districts in the United States are required to develop individual education programs (IEP) for every special-needs child. Some of the provisions of Public Law 94-142 are: developing an individualized plan specifying goals, objectives, and needed services for each child; allowance for as much time as possible spent in the mainstream classroom; the right of parents to be involved and to approve the IEP; lack of discrimination; protection of confidentiality and other provisions to ensure that your child receives a public education adequate to meet his or her needs.

New legislation in the past three years has tightened up some of the provisions of Public Law 94-142. Prior to this legislation, it was difficult to qualify ADD children as disabled under the law. Now, under the category "other health impaired" ADD children do qualify for special assistance if they have difficulty learning in a normal classroom.

If you or the school believe your child needs IEP assistance, it is a good idea to advocate on your child's behalf and participate in the development of the program. This will help him or her get the help required to develop basic learning skills.

In spite of legal requirements to see that your child gets the help he or she needs, some teachers are not comfortable dealing with ADD children. ADD children do disrupt class, fail to obey instructions, blurt out, will not remain seated, etc. All these behaviors are unsettling to the class. Teachers need to handle these disruptions along with educating a class of twenty to thirty children, which, of course, is asking a lot.

It is very important for you to work with your child's teacher, assisting him or her in helping your child. You do not need to be apologetic. It is sometimes difficult to balance the frustrations and limitations of your child's teacher with the needs of your child. Nevertheless, it is important to see that your child receives as much help as possible. The best way to do this is to maintain close contact with the teacher, offer help to resolve some of the problems, and keep the lines of communication open.

The problem does not end there, however. If your child's ADD behavior is troublesome to himself and classmates, additional interventions need to be made. The following material is presented as an aid to resolving some ADD problems that are intensified in a classroom setting.

PROBLEMS WITH FOCUSING

1. Check medication levels and schedules so that adequate biochemical balances are maintained during class time.
2. Have the teacher seat your child close by, ideally in the front row. If possible, try to surround your child with classmates who are both mature and good students.

3. When the teacher gives instructions, have him or her encourage your child to ask questions or repeat instructions if your child's mind appears to wander.

4. When possible, assign study teams so that your child is more involved with peers and more stimulated to stay alert when he or she is working with others.

5. Simplify, or break down into smaller parts, more complex instructions and assignments. Have the teacher explain instructions both orally and in writing. If necessary, have the child go to the teacher's desk quietly to ask for clarification of class instructions. If your child appears to be puzzled or lost, the teacher can ask the child to come forward for help.

6. Have the teacher develop cues to remind your child to refocus his or her attention. Sample cues might be giving finger signals that your child's mind is wandering. If the teacher notices that your child is not focused because his or her eyes are not on the assignment or appears not to be writing with the rest of the class, the teacher might call his or her name softly and lift a forefinger as a reminder to focus on the assignment. If the child is focusing and happens to look at the teacher, he or she can give the child another cue such as smiling or making a thumbs-up sign to indicate that he or she is pleased with your child's attentiveness.

   The teacher might also try checking on your child a given number of times during each period of study, making a check mark each time he or she finds the child focusing on work. At the end of the period, or at recess, the teacher could share the results with your child and encourage him or her to try to get more check marks. A more elaborate system would be to have the child bring the score home and set up a reward system for staying focused. The scorecard in the next chapter on homework problems could easily be adapted to this purpose.

7. Another focusing method is to use a monitoring tape to make a small noise every few minutes. The teacher makes a check mark each time the child is paying attention when the signal goes off. Older children can learn to monitor themselves with this method. Making such a tape is discussed in more detail in Chapter 15, "Easing the Homework Struggle."

   Once again, the scorecard discussed in Number 6 can be used to track results and set up a reward system.

8. When tests are given, the teacher can allow the child extra time to complete the assigned work.
9. The teacher can make some assignments shorter to coincide with your child's attention span.
10. A mentor student or peer assistant may be assigned to your child to help him or her organize work and study, and to help your child understand instructions and assignments.

These suggestions are designed to assist the teacher in being more helpful to your child. They may also trigger other ideas you or your child's teacher may have. Sometimes a combination of the above strategies needs to be applied. For children who have extreme difficulty remaining focused, a point chart and reward program such as the ones discussed in earlier chapters and mentioned in Number 6 can be helpful.

If focusing remains a serious problem after applying some of the suggestions presented here, it could be that your child may not be able to learn without a carefully structured special program designed to meet his or her needs. In such cases, you should consider intervening with the school and asking that an IEP be developed under the guidelines of the law described previously.

Keep in mind that your teacher's personal resources are limited; all of the above suggestions may not be practical. If you present the suggestion not as requirement, but as ideas to be considered to help your child manage his or her ADD problems, most teachers will appreciate your efforts and your thoughtful ideas.

HYPERACTIVITY AND IMPULSIVENESS

1. As previously mentioned, if your child is on medication it is important that it be taken at proper intervals so that he or she is receiving optimum benefit from it during class time. If your child is on a schedule that requires taking medication during the school day and this is not practical, you may want to ask your doctor about time-release medication.
2. Seat the child next to the teacher and seat close friends away from the child.

3. Ignore minor inappropriate behavior. This requires the teacher to be a little more relaxed in accepting behavior that might be slightly below grade-level standards. Frequently, a small compromise on this point can avoid creating a lot of the attention and stimulation that the ADD mind thrives on. Attention deficit children are disabled children; they are not just "cutups" or trying to get the best of the teacher. It is helpful if the teacher seeks support from the principal, parents, aids, and others who can be helpful in drawing a fair but softer line.

4. Allow the child to stand next to his or her desk if becoming too fidgety. An agreement can be prearranged so that the child will be allowed to stand if he or she has too much trouble sitting for long periods.

5. If the child has a tendency to blurt out answers, have the teacher make it clear that he or she will be called on only when his or her hand is raised. Then, if the child does blurt out an answer without being called upon, the teacher can ask the child if his or her hand was raised, as a reminder of proper procedures. The teacher should reinforce him or her with verbal praise when the child answers correctly.

6. Outside of class time, the teacher can develop a cue system with the child to help him or her be aware of becoming hyperactive or impulsive. Facial or hand expressions can be used as cues.

7. Instruct children seated near the ADD child to ignore hyperactive behavior. This reduces the reward the child otherwise receives for being disruptive.

8. In some circumstances, the teacher may be able to appoint one or two classmates to remind the child that he or she is beginning to act up.

9. If the child is disruptive and cannot show self-control, a time-out chair can be used in the classroom. The teacher should establish specific ground rules with the child ahead of time. The teacher might tell the child that if he or she begins to disrupt the class, a reminder will be used as an alert. If two reminders are given and the child continues to be disruptive, a time out will be warranted. If the teacher will follow an Awareness—Awareness—Choice model that is similar to the one you are using at home, the child will benefit from the consistency.

10. The teacher can experiment with allowing the child to monitor the time out so that the child chooses when to return to his or her seat. If this does not work, the teacher can give the child a time out of specific duration. Other choices might be to allow the child to stand beside his or her desk, or let the child make a choice between standing next to his or her desk or sitting in the time-out chair.

11. Some of the reward or point chart systems I mentioned in the previous section on managing distractibility can be used for the hyperactive child. Recording misbehavior and rewarding improvement frequently works reasonably well. Setting up behavior contracts and involving the parents in the reward system offers the child greater incentive for improvement.

ADDITIONAL NOTES

Organization

Many children with ADD have problems organizing their desks, which adds to their difficulties in keeping up with schoolwork. They lose papers, cannot find books, misplace assignments, and in general have messy, unorganized desks. This slows them down in the classroom. When the teacher is reading from a text, they cannot find the text, or they cannot find the page of the text because they were frantically looking for the book while instructions were being given.

Teaching organization skills to these children is important. They need to know where to look to find materials that are being used in class. If the teacher demonstrates desk organization to the class and follows up with the children who have trouble in this area, some of these problems improve. An alternate method is to have another student assigned to help the ADD child find the needed material and/or the place in the assignment that is being used in class. Most children with organizational problems benefit from spending a few minutes with the teacher or a mentor at the end of class to prepare their desk for the next day.

Study Skills

Many ADD children are weak in the following areas:

1. Understanding the key ideas in study material
2. Remembering the main points of the assignment
3. Prioritizing information that has been learned
4. Understanding instructions given by the teacher
5. Breaking down longer assignments into shorter assignments and allocating time to complete projects

This list is not complete, but it suggests that ADD children need help to strengthen their study skills. Taking notes, making lists of important material to remember, and asking themselves why some material is important can be helpful to ADD children. Some of the ideas presented in Chapter 15 on homework problems offer help in strengthening weak study skills.

Teaching study skills is very important. Initially the teacher might be able to help strengthen your child's study skills. An IEP will address many problems. If your child does not qualify for an IEP, you may need to call upon other resources. You yourself may want to take over this tutoring. Perhaps a schoolmate can demonstrate how he or she studies and help your child build skills. If this is not possible, hiring a private tutor might be a consideration.

Your child may have a specific learning disability along with ADD that prevents him or her from making progress in schoolwork. A number of excellent learning centers and tutors are available in most areas to help your child with special needs.

The more these technical problems can be resolved the easier it will be for your child to perform better in class. Learning effective study skills will pay dividends at school, doing homework, and in building self-esteem.

A FINAL WORD

Most ADD children experience at least some school or homework problems. These challenges are important, to be sure. But sometimes these problems are allowed to overshadow others that are of equal or greater significance. It is important to remember that as your child moves toward adulthood, one day his or her school years will be left behind. However, the struggle to meet the demands of daily life will continue.

I believe that character formation, developing a sense of self-esteem, and the ability to reassure oneself when challenges arise are extremely important traits to have. For this reason, I place more immediate emphasis on controlling aggressive impulses, temper tantrums, and other types of negative behavior patterns than on difficulties that are specific to the school environment. Ultimately, if a child is held back a grade while his or her class moves ahead, or if he or she requires special teaching, the discomfort of these experiences will pass. Education is very important to your child's development, but, like everything else, it needs to be kept in perspective.

Chapter 15

Easing the Homework Struggle

"There's no use trying," she said, "one can't believe impossible things." "I dare say you haven't had much practice," said the Queen. "When I was your age, I always did it for half-an-hour a day."

Lewis Carroll
The Walrus and the Carpenter

Many ADD children find homework overwhelming. The difficulty of getting started on unpleasant tasks rears its head when homework time comes around as the child faces many of his or her shortcomings all at once. Forgetfulness, incomprehension, lack of interest, difficulty remaining seated, trouble focusing, boredom, and inability to organize or to break down assignments into smaller units are a few of the many reasons ADD children will do as much as they can to avoid homework.

The discomforts of telling a few white lies, purposely misunderstanding assignments, and being nagged or reprimanded by parents are small prices to pay for avoiding that which is dreaded.

I remember my own struggle as an ADD child, finally sitting down to study, just to get it over with because the pressure from my father was unbearable. I would read a page or two and Dad would come in and question me on what I read. I could not answer because I did not remember the material, which would lead to more incrimination. Finally Dad would read with me, then question me again—the results would not be much better. Holding my mind steady long enough to read two pages was a real challenge for me.

My brother was three years younger and quite a scholar. He would come home with two hours of regular homework along with extra-credit projects. I would report that I did not have homework, or that I just had a few minutes of work that was not very important. This incongruity between my brother's homework assignments and mine put me in a very weak bargaining position.

Each ADD child approaches homework with his or her own set of obstacles and challenges. I believe it is helpful for parents to understand why some tasks are especially difficult for their own child.

Since homework difficulties can cover a wide variety of issues, the best way to help children with homework is to gather as much information as possible on the underlying problems. To do this, use a checklist. The checklist then serves as a focal point for addressing particular problems your child is having. It will also help you understand how your child's ADD symptoms make homework such a chore, and allows you to help your child compensate for those weaknesses.

HELPING YOUR CHILD

The following checklist includes most of the problems I have encountered with homework assignments.

My child:

_____ does not write down the assignment when it is given at school

_____ does copy the assignment, but does not understand it

_____ copies and understands the assignment, but misplaces it

_____ forgets necessary books and materials

_____ postpones starting homework at home

_____ plays, daydreams, doodles, etc., but does not study at home

_____ rushes through work so that work is messy, illegible, etc.

_____ does not check for errors, is careless, makes many mistakes

_____ gets up every few minutes to go to the bathroom, blow his or her nose, etc.

_____ tries to study, but gets easily distracted, has trouble focusing, etc.

_____ studies, but does not retain much information, particularly when reading

_____ fails to turn in completed homework assignments

_____ other homework problems not stated above

Doing homework can be quite a complicated task, as this checklist shows. Many parents do not take this into consideration and think that by forcing their child to study in his or her room the problem is pretty much solved.

The first step in helping your child overcome homework difficulties is to use the above checklist or one like it to identify his or her study problems. Unless your child is just starting first grade, you probably already know some of the problems he or she is facing. However, you need to obtain more information than what is immediately obvious. This might include habits such as leaving books at school or forgetting to turn in assignments. Spend some time with your child as he or she studies to find out if he or she spends most study time playing or doodling. Does the child have trouble understanding the material? Does he or she have trouble retaining what has been studied? After you have compiled your information, you are ready to seek ways to help. Do not be too concerned about obtaining 100 percent of the information on the first try; as you work with your child and resolve the problems you uncover, other problems may emerge.

COMMUNICATING WITH YOUR CHILD'S TEACHER

Talk to your child's teacher about any study problems you have found. And do not worry that this might embarrass your child or you. You are much better off if you target the problems and let the teacher know what you know—what you do to help your child concentrate, ways you have found that work best to get your child to pay attention, etc. If your child is to enjoy even moderate success you need to see yourself as a cooperative partner with your child's teacher. Teachers are usually eager to help you and your child. They appreciate your interest and ideas.

If you can bring helpful ideas to parent/teacher meetings, such as the checklist and charts suggested in this chapter, your child's teacher will appreciate your effort. Many teachers already have methods of working with ADD children that are effective, but they do need your cooperation. Ask them how you can help. Volunteer your full participation. Teachers are always looking for better ways to manage challenging situations.

If your child is having problems at school as well as difficulty with homework, it is important that you communicate with your child's teacher to let him or her know what efforts you are making. Brainstorm ideas with her. Chapter 14, "How to Help Your Child with School," provides more information and guidelines on working with your child's teacher.

The following section outlines ways to help your child. Many of the interventions have been collected from my experiences working with teachers and children. Other sources that were helpful were the checklists from CHADD (Children and Adults with Attention Deficit Disorders) as well as Harvey C. Parker's book, *The ADD Hyperactivity Workbook.*

INTERVENTIONS

I. Child Does Not Write Down the Assignment When in School

1. The parent provides a worksheet listing each subject.
2. The child writes down the homework assignment for each subject on the worksheet.
3. The child shows the worksheet to the teacher who approves or corrects it.
4. The teacher agrees to ask the child for his or her worksheet each day.
5. The worksheet includes space for the teacher to comment on any incomplete assignments from the previous day.

This procedure should minimize difficulties such as the child forgetting or misunderstanding homework assignments. It also benefits

the child by helping him or her to assume responsibility for participating in the resolution of the problem.

Occasionally, problems may arise using this method. For example, your
child tells you he or she has lost the worksheet. Should this be the case, I
suggest that the parent provide the teacher with a self-addressed, stamped
envelope to mail you the daily assignments on a weekly basis. Examples of
daily and weekly worksheets follow. (See Figures 15.1 and 15.2.)

FIGURE 15.1. Daily Homework Sheet

MONDAY HOMEWORK SHEET	
Math	
Science	
English	
Other	
Teacher's approval/notes/comments:	

FIGURE 15.2. Weekly Homework Sheet

Weekly Homework: Week of _____					
Subject	Mon	Tues	Wed	Thurs	Fri
Math					
Science					
English					
Other					
Teacher's comments					

II. Child Copies the Assignment but Does Not Understand It

1. If you and your child are using the previous two worksheets to help remember homework, the teacher can explain the assignment to the child when the worksheet is presented, or use it to write a note to the parent explaining the work to be done. If your child does not need the above aids, he or she may do quite well simply asking the teacher to explain the homework assignments at the end of each school day.

2. An arrangement is made ahead of time with a specific child in your child's class who will act as a backup. You can then call that student to get information on homework assignments. If old enough, your child takes responsibility for himself or herself.
3. While in school, your child can get help from a mentor classmate designated by the teacher for this purpose.
4. Using a weekly homework assignment sheet such as the one in Figure 15.2, review assignments with your child. At the beginning of the week if there are questions, the parent can be prepared in advance and have time to make appropriate contacts.
5. If your child has trouble understanding the assignment during home study time and the above steps have been taken, you can help answer questions.

III. Child Copies and Understands the Assignment, But Misplaces It

1. Provide the child with a colored folder to hold assignment sheets and homework notes.
2. The teacher checks with the student to make sure the homework assignment is in the take-home folder.
3. The parent provides the teacher with a self-addressed stamped envelope in which to mail homework assignments for the following week.
4. If your child is still missing assignments, talk to a prearranged "backup" student to obtain the assignments.
5. Get the teacher's permission to call her for missing assignments, should these methods occasionally fail.
6. Some teachers have their class assignments listed on their voice mail at school. Check with your child's school to see if your child's teacher uses voice mail.

IV. Child Forgets Necessary Books and Materials

1. Purchase a second set of books to keep at home.
2. As the teacher is checking the homework assignment, he or she has your child show him or her the books that the child needs to bring home.

3. In lieu of buying a second set of books, if the child fails to bring home necessary study materials as suggested above, have him or her carry all books home every night. This will usually prompt the child to "remember" so that he or she can carry a lighter load.
4. If occasionally one book is forgotten call the backup student and see if the book may be borrowed for a few hours.

V. Child Postpones Starting His or Her Homework at Home

1. Check to make sure medication levels are okay. Many children take one dosage in the morning and one at noon. Frequently when children sit down to study in the late afternoon or early evening, they are no longer benefiting from the earlier dosage. If you think this may be a problem, check with your child's doctor.
2. Start homework study at the same time every day.
3. Allow your child to relax and unwind for approximately one half hour after arriving home from school.
4. Implement a policy of "STUDY FIRST THEN PLAY." When homework is completed your child earns the privilege of playing with friends, watching television, having free time, etc.
5. If, over a period of time, your child shows that he or she is acting responsibly and getting homework done before play, then explore other study times. If procrastination starts all over again, shift back to "STUDY FIRST THEN PLAY."
6. BE CONSTANT AND UNWAVERING WHEN AWARDING FREE TIME (Number 4).
7. Compliment your child frequently on the successful completion of homework.

VI. Child Plays, Daydreams, Doodles, etc., but Does Not Study at Home

1. This can be a clear indication that medication dosages need to be adjusted. Reread Number 1 in intervention V.
2. Do not allow radio, television, siblings, or any other distractions in your child's study area.

3. Be sure to enforce the "STUDY FIRST THEN PLAY" policy.

4. Ask your child if he or she is having trouble understanding the material or thinks it is too difficult. If this is the case, help your child to understand the assignment but do not do the homework for him or her.

5. Allow your child brief breaks from studying to work off excess energy, particularly if he or she has trouble sitting quietly or fidgets and squirms in other situations. A seven-year-old child might be able to sit for fifteen to twenty minutes. Older children, ages ten to twelve, can usually last more than thirty minutes. Three-minute breaks to stretch, walk around the room, go to the bathroom, or get a glass of water should be sufficient.

6. Use a timer to help your child meet specific study time goals. After fifteen minutes of studying the child earns a break. Once you set the timer, if the child doodles or daydreams for more than a minute or two, that time is added on to the end of the study period before a break is allowed.

7. You can also make a tape with a monitoring sound such as a clang or beep that sounds every minute. If your child tends to daydream the sound on the tape can bring him or her back to the task at hand. More detail on how to use a monitoring tape is given in intervention X.

8. During the child's study time, check on him or her every ten or twelve minutes. If you find your child at work, reward him or her with congratulations or by giving bonus points. You can also set up a simple reward system for children up to age eleven, congratulating them or giving them points when you check on them if they are studying. If study time is one hour, five or six ten- or-twelve-minute checks give them the opportunity to earn a reward for staying on their task. More detail on setting this up is given in intervention X.

VII. *Child Rushes Through Work; Work Is Messy, Illegible, etc.*

1. This problem is very common with ADD children. They are far more likely to have illegible handwriting and a general ten-

dency toward messiness. I suggest parents and teachers give some leeway in this area.

Place your emphasis on general learning rather than on neatness. Encourage improvement in neatness but do not press for perfection. Homework needs to be readable but use discretion about making a fuss over smudges and the like. The child will perceive rewriting homework when it is not really necessary as punishment. Push too hard for neatness and your ADD child will get discouraged.

2. The desire to get unpleasant tasks over with quickly will cause the ADD child to rush through homework. This can also produce poor handwriting. When you check the homework to see that the work is completed allow some leeway with handwriting and neatness, but make sure it is legible.

3. When you are enforcing the "STUDY FIRST THEN PLAY" rule the child may be inclined to rush through homework to play with friends. If this is happening and one hour of homework is completed in twenty-five minutes, you will need to set a time period for study. If the child is using a homework sheet to keep track of assignments, the teacher can indicate approximately how long the assignment should take. You can then use this time estimate as the minimum amount of time the child is required to do homework. Frequently, talking with other parents on an informal basis can give you a good idea of how long homework generally takes. Setting a time period will usually help lessen the problem of rushing through work.

VIII. *Child Does Not Check for Errors,*
Is Careless, Makes Many Mistakes

1. This problem is very common with ADD children. Their propensity to finish low-motivation tasks quickly plus their desire to engage in activities that are more appealing will motivate them to speed through homework.

   As discussed previously, the best solution to this problem is to allocate a specific period of time to complete homework. This tends to eliminate any value in rushing to get to playtime. I also suggest that an additional ten minutes or so be added to the end of the study period to review errors and mistakes. After some initial coaching, you can turn some of the responsibility of correcting mistakes over to your child. At the end of the study period ask the child to do a ten-minute review and show you the corrections he or she made. The importance of the extra time is that the child learns to review his or her work before showing it to you or presenting it to the teacher.

2. Some of the problems with errors and incompleteness stem from weak focusing ability. If this appears to be a factor with your child you may want to employ some of the techniques discussed in intervention X.

IX. Child Gets Up Every Few Minutes to Go to the Bathroom, Answer the Telephone, Look Out the Window, etc.

1. I like to remedy this problem by setting brief (three-minute) breaks every fifteen to twenty minutes depending on the age of the child. A three-minute walk around the room is enough time to burn off energy or to go to the bathroom.
2. No outside interference should be permitted during study time. Incoming telephone calls can be answered after homework is completed. It is important to set the rules of study ahead of time.

X. Child Tries to Study, but Gets Easily Distracted, Has Trouble Focusing, etc.

1. The challenge here is to beat distractions. Your child's mind will drift at times. In spite of the attempts your child makes to manage this challenge, his or her mind will still drift, daydream, or get lost in thought. A resolution not to do this is generally not sufficient to stop what I sometimes call "the swivel head syndrome."
2. Expect some mental wandering, particularly if your child is making an effort to study. Allow your child a little slack in this area.
3. Medication can help your child focus. When your child starts homework make sure that he or she is gaining the benefits of medication. As mentioned above, if your child's last medication was around noontime, and he or she is starting to study at

4:00 p.m. he or she is most likely working without the benefit of medication.

This is one reason I like to see children study in the afternoon or, if they prove they can avoid homework problems, early in the evening. Check with your doctor to be sure that the medication and dosing sequences are effective.

4. The best way to manage distractibility is to make your child aware that it is happening. As the child is made aware that he or she is drifting, attention can be drawn back to the assignment at hand.

5. As mentioned in intervention VI, you will have to employ some kind of stimulus arousal. I like using a tape that will remind the child to return to study. Generally it is a good idea to observe your child studying to see how frequently his or her mind drifts. Older children usually have a better ability to stay focused longer than younger children do.

I suggest you purchase a sixty-minute audiotape for this purpose. As you record on the tape make sure there are no extraneous sounds and that the background is quiet. Every sixty seconds, make a sound on the tape. Any clean sound will do. With your watch handy, gently strike a metal or glass bowl with a spoon every sixty seconds. Do this throughout the entire tape. On the reverse side of the tape, do the same but this time at intervals of ninety seconds.

When your child begins to study, turn on the tape player. Tell your child that the periodic sounds are reminders to keep his or her attention on study. For the first few sessions it would be a good idea to spend the study period with your child to see if he or she does it, or if you need to remind your child what the sound is for. This method generally works well. If your child's mind drifts a lot, the signal every sixty seconds will minimize his or her daydreaming or at least make the child more aware of the need to focus.

6. Another method you can employ is to check on your child randomly. If your child is not too distractible, or if he or she has gained focusing skills using the audiotape, you may want to make ten to fifteen random checks during a study period. Vary the intervals so that sometimes you check after a two- or three-

minute period and other times after ten or fifteen minutes. You could make up a reward chart to score your child's results.

The idea is that a perfect score could be obtained if your child is attentive each time you check. Using a fifteen-check focusing scorecard (see Figure 15.3), fifteen would equal 100 percent, twelve would equal 80 percent, nine would equal 70 percent, and so forth. You might want to chart your child's progress and offer some incentive or small reward for improvement. Remember, ADD children thrive on positive strokes!

XI. Child Studies, But Does Not Retain Information, Particularly When Reading

1. This problem is fed by many ADD characteristics. If you have taken appropriate steps to increase your child's motivation, set a fixed period of time for study to reduce hurriedness, removed distractions, dealt with fidgeting, and managed the problems your child has that have been discussed above, you are ready to help your child comprehend his or her homework.

   Frequently, difficulties in performing one or more of the following three processes contribute to your child's inability to assimilate reading material: *prioritizing information, understanding information,* and *remembering.*

XII. Child Has a Problem Prioritizing Information

This deals with selecting the main or principal ideas in the reading material, discarding background material, and focusing on important ideas. If your child tries to understand and retain *everything* he or she reads, with no concept of what is important, the child will simply be overwhelmed by the task.

1. To determine if this is a problem, select a small reading assignment and ask your child what the important points of the article are. Try this with various assignments because comprehension can vary depending upon the contents of the material. For instance, select an article on a subject your child is very interested in or that he or she knows well. Ask your child to read it and tell you what is important. He or she should be able to select many of

FIGURE 15.3. Focusing Scorecard

Focusing Scorecard					
	Mon	Tues	Wed	Thurs	Fri
1					
2					
3					
4					
5					
6					
7					
8					
9					
10					
11					
12					
13					
14					
15					
Total					

the main points. Examples of such readings vary with age. Very young children might want to hear the fairy tale of *The Three Little Pigs*. They should be able to point out that the safety of the pigs was very important, and that the brick house was a very important idea. Older children like to play video games. After reading the game's instructions they should be able to tell you what is important and what is background material.

2. Use sample reading material as a way of introducing the idea that not all writing is of equal importance. Discuss the difference between what is important and what is not. Review a few examples of materials your child is familiar with to be sure he or she understands the concept. This is knowledge that your child will use for the rest of his or her life.

3. Once you have acquainted your child with the concept of prioritizing information, take simple ideas from his or her assignments. You can begin by asking questions that the child might regard as silly. "What was the flavor of tea that was thrown overboard at the Boston Tea Party?" "When George Washington crossed the Delaware, was it important that he rode in a particular type of boat?" Ask him or her why the flavor of the tea or type of boat is not important.

4. Return to his or her homework assignment. Break the reading down to one page at a time. Ask the child to read a page and tell you what was important. For example, the purpose of the Boston Tea Party and its historical significance are important; the flavor of the tea is not. Similarly, why Washington crossed the Delaware is more important than how many people were in the boat with him. You may have to spend some time with your child at first and repeat the same question several times. When your child finishes the assignment he or she should have a better understanding of prioritizing information.

5. An index card with a question on it can be a constant reminder to look for the important material. Each time your child begins homework, have him or her read a page, then pause and ask what he or she just read and what is most important to remember. The question the child wants to learn and apply is "What are the most important ideas on this page?"

XIII. Child Has a Problem Understanding Information

Understanding requires us to grasp the meaning of what we have read and organize that information in a sequential fashion. If you have worked with your child to help him or her prioritize written material, you are ready to teach your child some simple tools for increasing comprehension.

The key to increasing your child's comprehension lies in understanding and enhancing the way your child thinks. Thinking is enhanced when, in addition to prioritizing information, your child can *summarize* and *explain* (using his or her own words) the meaning of what he or she has read.

You can help your child by having him or her read aloud, underline words that are important, make brief notes, use index cards to summarize the information, and explain to you what he or she has studied. Teach your child that difficult chapters of a book can be outlined to make them more comprehensible. What we are discussing here is basic note-taking skills that every college student is acquainted with. Your child is not too young to develop good study habits. Your coaching in the initial stages will be very important, so approach this teaching with utmost patience. You may wish to make up a simple study sheet (see Figure 15.4) to help your child with homework. This sheet can be used to review studied material at test time.

FIGURE 15.4. Study Sheet

History Pages: _____
Key Points:
What This Means to Me:

You may find that your child could benefit from some tutoring. Ask your child's teacher if there is a student he or she can recommend as a tutor. Discuss strategies with the tutor and focus on study strengths you would like to see your child develop.

XIV. Child Fails to Turn in Completed Homework Assignments

1. Make sure your child leaves for school in the morning with his or her homework sheets.
2. Put the homework in his or her colorful homework folder.
3. If permitted, make a colorful sign for your child's school desk that reads "Turn in Assignment."
4. Notify your child's teacher that this is a problem and ask him or her to ask your child for the assignment.
5. If your child is having the teacher check his or her homework assignment sheet before leaving for the day, ask the teacher to collect the previous day's homework at that time.

The above ideas should help your child improve homework assignments and perform better in school. Should you apply these techniques and find your child is not making progress, discuss this with your therapist or schoolteacher. Your child may have a specific learning disability. If you believe this may be the case, you can have your child tested by the school to determine if this is so. Special classes are set up specifically to tutor children with learning disabilities.

Attention deficit disorder is recognized as a disability. If the individual needs of ADD children cannot be met in a normal class, they are entitled under Public Law 94-142 to be placed in a program that provides special services. Information on this process is discussed in Chapter 14 of this book, "How to Help Your Child with School."

Chapter 16

Peers and Socialization

How does it feel
To be on your own
With no direction . . .
Like a complete unknown
Like a rolling stone

Bob Dylan
"Like a Rolling Stone"

RELATIONSHIP PROBLEMS

If you are the parent of an ADD child you will certainly be aware of the difficulties that ADD children have with children their own age. It is important to realize that ADD children are not aware of the effects that their actions have on other people. When playing with others, the same traits that cause them difficulty at home or at school are sometimes compounded because other children are uncomfortable with their behavior. To be sure, inattentiveness, impulsiveness, hyperactivity, and emotional volatility translate into behavior that is either frightening or off-putting to the very children they want to play with.

If ADD children are aggressive, bossy, will not take turns, cry easily, and only think of themselves, they may find they are left out of many play activities. Understandably, this leads ADD children to become needy, desperately seeking someone to play with. This very neediness tends to drive other children farther away from them; as a result, the ADD child becomes even more demanding and clinging.

Other times, the forced isolation by peers may cause your child to withdraw and give up, frustrated and fearing rejection. It is not unusual to see ADD children bounce between these two extremes—frustrated and angry one moment, filled with fear of rejection the next.

These problems tend to be exacerbated with age because the child's social skills do not develop at the same rate as those of his or her peers. What is more, as relationships become more subtle and complex, the ADD child's inability to keep up causes him or her to feel increasingly isolated.

It is important to remember that social interaction is complex no matter who we are. In fact, many adults have difficulty mastering different social situations. Part of the problem young children face is that no clear-cut guidelines for learning social behavior exist as there are for learning to read, write, or add numbers. For the most part children are not taught how to play. It is simply assumed that they will learn it naturally.

I think it would be a good idea in the early primary school grades to have a short time each week devoted to teaching play skills. It would help all children with more highly developed social skills to be more compassionate and patient with their peers, whatever range of skills their peers might have. And it would certainly help those children with ADD develop skills that would make them more acceptable to their peers.

Social interaction requires a good deal of awareness of other people. For instance, many interactions are nonverbal. To understand the nonverbal cues, we must be attentive to others and control our own responses. Both are tasks that many ADD children find extremely difficult.

Another problem is that once your child gets off to a bad start with his or her peers, it is very difficult to live down that reputation. The child's troublesome behavior easily brands him or her as difficult or at least different.

Children can be cruel, no doubt about it. Those who are different are not only left out of play, but are frequently made the brunt of jokes and are the continual target of pranks, taunting, and bullying.

I have had many parents tell me that their children were not safe at school or after school because other children would threaten them or beat them up. Many parents change schools to give their children a fresh start, only to see the same cycle repeat itself.

Bear in mind that learning to make friends and develop play skills can be one of your ADD child's biggest challenges. Any child with weak social skills has a difficult road ahead. As parents, we are understandably eager to have our children make friends and enjoy playing with others. First and foremost, if you are to help your child you will need to accept modest gains from him or her, gains that sometimes come at a maddeningly slow pace. There is no easy or quick method to accelerate social development.

A SOCIAL SKILLS MODEL

The following model suggests some of the skills that are required for good social interaction.

Communication

Your child needs to learn how to

1. Introduce himself or herself to others appropriately
2. Enter an ongoing conversation unobtrusively
3. Start a conversation when appropriate
4. Interrupt a conversation courteously
5. Answer questions when asked
6. Show gratitude
7. Learn how to compliment others
8. Give positive feedback when asked for comments on the successes and good news of others
9. Not accuse others when something goes wrong
10. Not blame others
11. Be able to keep quiet while others talk and show alert listening skills
12. Encourage others to talk about what they want
13. Accept criticism graciously
14. Acknowledge mistakes and "goof ups" humorously, if possible
15. Share, wait, or take turns in the conversation
16. Handle being teased
17. Apologize when appropriate
18. Not talk too much and avoid bragging
19. Disagree without criticizing or putting others down
20. Leave the group or individual discussion in a timely fashion and develop good "good-bye" skills

Nonverbal Skills

Your child should be taught to

1. Make eye contact
2. Keep appropriate physical distance
3. Smile, nod, and make other facial expressions appropriately
4. Contain emotions—does not cry or get too upset
5. Avoid touching others except when rarely called for
6. Look for subtle body and facial cues in others and interpret them correctly
7. Laugh and/or respond as the general group does

Emotional Control

Your child may need help to

1. Handle peer pressure in social settings without getting upset
2. Resist blurting out, making inappropriate remarks, or hurting others
3. Identify his or her own emotions and express them appropriately— be able to say, "I'm angry," or "I'm feeling frustrated," etc.
4. Avoid crying
5. Control his or her temper
6. Contain his or her anger rather than shouting or screaming
7. Contain impulsiveness and understand that being bossy or domineering will not endear him or her to others
8. Develop an ability to focus on others rather than being self-absorbed
9. Wait his or her turn to talk, play, etc.
10. Not quit a game before it is over, or take his or her playthings away before the end of play
11. Follow rules or instructions of play, watching or asking questions if not sure

Winning Friends

Teach your child to

1. Ask others what they want to do
2. Encourage others to do what they want

3. Give compliments
4. Offer to help
5. Compromise and develop skills to work out conflicts fairly
6. Accept "no" for an answer without begging or badgering others to change
7. Share snacks and other items
8. Ask others if they like what they are doing, or if they want to change the game or play
9. Ask if others are having a good time
10. Verbalize his or her enjoyment in playing with the others
11. Do small favors

These lists are by no means complete. However, they do give you an idea where your child's skills need to be strengthened or expanded. The checklist provides you with an opportunity to identify areas to focus on and then make clear choices about where to begin.

Use a highlighter to mark the skills your child lacks. If you find that your child is weak in all the areas, which is not unusual, do not be alarmed. Having identified the problem areas, pick one or two places where you are first going to put your time and energy.

Watch your child play and go through the list again after making your observations. From time to time, monitor your child's play so you can reaffirm the skills you checked. Prioritize the areas you think are the most seriously in need of your coaching. Even if you check most of the items on the list, you may observe that your child's skills in some areas are stronger than in others. You may find that your child can manage certain skills some of the time but is completely lacking in others. As you concentrate your efforts in one area or another, try not to worry about those areas you are neglecting for now. Most of the principles behind developing good relationships are pretty much contained in the golden rule—"Treat other people as you would liked to be treated." Almost all of the items on the previous lists come down to that. Once your child truly grasps the concept in one area, it will spill over into others.

Figure 16.1 contains a short list for your child's teacher to complete. Incorporate his or her information with your observations in prioritizing your list.

To prioritize the list, mark each of your highlighted skills with a 1, 2, or 3. A 3 indicates a skill that you identify as important, to be

FIGURE 16.1. Social Questionnaire: Teacher Form

Child's Name _____   Teacher's Name _____

Indicate whether the child has a social interaction problem by circling the appropriate interaction number(s) on the left. Review the list a second time, numbering the circled interactions with a 1, 2, or 3 in the blank on the right. Entering 1 indicates a lesser problem with that social skill; entering 2 indicates a moderate problem; entering 3 indicates a high degree of frequency or severity with that social skill.

   1. Rough—hits, pushes, shoves others   _____
   2. Grabby   _____
   3. Bossy   _____
   4. Dominates activities   _____
   5. Intrudes in others' games   _____
   6. Quits a game before it is completed   _____
   7. Has trouble waiting his or her turn   _____
   8. Does not pay attention to the game; does not know what to do   _____
   9. Talks too much   _____
  10. Does not listen to others   _____
  11. Blames or accuses others in the game   _____
  12. Insensitive to the feelings of others   _____
  13. Too focused on self   _____
  14. Misses nonverbal cues   _____
  15. Unable to share or participate in give and take   _____
  16. Loses temper   _____
  17. Loses emotional control (cries easily, displays anger, etc.)   _____
  18. Is needy, clingy, dependent on others   _____
  19. Is afraid of participating, fears making mistakes or being
      rejected   _____
  20. Trouble with the following communication skills
      in conversation (nonplay)   _____
      a. Does not enter ongoing conversation easily   _____
      b. Interrupts others   _____
      c. Does not listen when others speak   _____
      d. Criticizes, blames, or accuses others   _____
      e. Misses nonverbal communication cues   _____
      f. Pesters others   _____
      g. Has trouble handling teasing or joking   _____
      h. Does not laugh, speak, or respond as the general group
          does   _____

worked on immediately. A 2 indicates skills that are important but not of highest priority. Number 1 skills are those in which your child has shown some mastery and/or skills that are not of high priority that are to be developed last.

Before we proceed with the next section let me remind you that you will be striving to make small gains. The biggest mistake most parents make is to attempt too much change at one time. This overloads the child and is a setup for failure. It will take a lot of effort to teach very rudimentary skills, so do not set yourself or your child up for disappointment. Improvement will come slowly and only with a lot of practice.

Your child's teacher can also provide information on social strengths and weaknesses. The Social Questionnaire teacher form can be used to obtain more precise information from school sources.

COACHING YOUR CHILD

As you combine the information from your own checklist with that of the school, you can decide on the one area that you want to work on first. The following questions suggest some social skills you may want to initially focus on:

Decide on the Skill Area You Wish to Teach

- Do you want to help your child initiate contact with a peer and begin a conversation?
- Do you want to help your child maintain a conversation by listening and responding better?
- Do you wish to help your child become aware of an ongoing conversation or play activity and join in appropriately?
- Do you want to teach your child to be aware of subtle nonverbal cues?
- Do you want to teach your child to manage his or her emotions?
- Do you want to teach your child to handle teasing and baiting?
- Do you want to teach your child to ask questions, be sure others are enjoying themselves, and be attentive to others?
- Do you want to teach your child not to be bossy or try to control play and conversation?

- Do you want to help your child contain his or her neediness?
- Do you want to teach your child the art of sharing?
- Do you want to teach your child how to make compromises, accept criticism, and stop accusing others?
- Do you want to help your child to play without roughhousing, becoming too wild or too highly "revved"?

Once you have narrowed down the skill area you wish to teach, you will need to define it clearly and explain the individual components of social interaction that it involves. Make a checklist of the key components for your child to see and work with. If you are teaching your child to listen and respond to conversations, a checklist might look like this:

_____ Be aware and listen. What was just said?
_____ Allow the other person to complete what he or she wanted to say.
_____ Ask a few questions to clarify, when appropriate.
_____ Be aware of, and hold back, your urge to complete other people's sentences or blurt out words.
_____ Talk without bragging.
_____ Do not tire others by talking too much.
_____ Encourage and/or compliment others as appropriate.
_____ Show genuine interest with exclamation when appropriate.
_____ Say, "Whoops, I missed what you said," when your mind drifts and attention lapses.
_____ Learn to disagree without putting other people down.

As you make a list and practice with your child, you will find through practice and observation that your child does other things which make him or her a poor conversationalist. For example, the child looks around the room when someone is talking to him or her. Add these observations to your list.

You are now ready to practice some basic social skills. If the list is long, then practice a smaller section. Start by working on just a few skills.

- Model the skill you want to teach.
- Act out the skill with your child.

- Critique (point out to your child the mistakes he or she makes in practicing the skill).
- Role-play again.
- Practice frequently.
- Engage spouse, sibling, or others in role-playing. For example, if you are teaching your child to pay attention, one spouse can ignore the other while the second spouse can share how upset he is because he feels rejected.
- Make the role-play more challenging as skills develop.
- Observe your child practicing with another child.
- Critique the role-play.
- Role-play situations you have critiqued.
- Review the components of the skill area you have defined and ask your child to solve difficult problems from among those components.
- Continue practicing as you mix and match the list.
- Continue to work on the area you have chosen until some of the new skills become a habit. Do not move too fast to another problem area or your child will lose much or all of what he or she has learned.

ENTERING THE SOCIAL ARENA

Supervised Play at Home

As you begin to work with your child, keep it as simple as you can. For example, invite one child at a time to your house to play. ADD children are better with a single playmate than with groups. And if you have only your own child and one other child to watch, it is going to be relatively easy to monitor your child's play skills.

You will probably find that your ADD child will do best with a playmate one or two years younger than himself.

You can help your child by limiting the amount of time he or she spends with friends. Do not let the children play for long periods without supervision. It is best to invite a child to spend one or two hours at your house. Plan interesting things for the children to do. You can arrange for the children to watch a video, play a computer game, do some crafts together, or help you with a project that will involve them and be within their skill and interest levels. Serve snacks; all children like tasty snacks, and you can be present during snack time to help with social conversation.

If you select activities the children enjoy, serve snacks, and keep the visits short, children may begin to regard your child's house as a fun place to be.

Supervised Play on Outings

Scheduling trips with a friend on the weekend is another way your child can enjoy company his or her age and develop skills under your supervision. Going to the beach, a movie, the zoo, the playground, to see a parade, or anything children would consider interesting can be a sure hit with your guest.

Such activities allow you to supervise and observe your child in a social context, while providing enough structure to keep social interaction positive and constructive.

Supervised Play in the Community

Community activities where there is a lot of adult supervision and structure are the best opportunities to ease your child into group situations. Certain team sports, church groups, hobby groups, scouts, or programs run by your local recreation department offer supervised group activities. Other activities might be offered by your local YMCA, exercise and dance classes, or children's martial arts classes, to mention a few. Be prepared to help your child build his or her social skills in order to participate in these activities.

School Play

School play is the most difficult arena for your child to develop skills. Some children never master the skills necessary to enjoy recess or lunchtime with peers, where free play provides plenty of opportunities for teasing and bullying, which most ADD kids do not handle well.

Sometimes a teacher or principal can ask a socially sophisticated mentor student to take your child under his or her wing. The mentor looks after your child and protects him or her from groups that would give your child a difficult time. Other times, the mentor plays with your child one on one, and may invite one or two other mature children to play as well.

I have seen this method work and I like to suggest it. Not many schools attempt to do this and I hope to encourage parents to bring the idea to their own child's school.

Your support is of vital importance. Keep working with your child's skill development. The best your child might manage may be to gain a few younger friends that he or she can play with at school. Encourage those friendships while you explore other ways to help your child enrich friendships and expand social contacts.

It is important to let your child's teacher know that he or she has problems on the playground. This information can be communicated to the playground supervisor, who can keep an eye out to prevent bullying and other forms of aggressive teasing.

Alternative Ways to Help Your Child

If your child continues to have severe social problems in the public school system and you are able to afford a private school, I suggest you consider this option. Many small private schools are prepared to manage the social problems we have discussed.

Other alternatives include finding a children's therapy group that offers social skills counseling. This is an excellent way to have your child meet other children and gain social awareness. If you cannot find such a group, you may want to seek the help of a professional who works with children and can tailor an individual program to help your child.

Chapter 17

Daily Challenges
and How to Meet Them

The act of being wise is the art of knowing what to overlook.

William James
The Principles of Psychology

You are likely to encounter a number of problems with your child that can be solved without the more elaborate point charts and techniques we used to manage the more serious behaviors discussed in earlier chapters.

For the most part, the use of natural consequences (discussed in Chapter 5) will be sufficient to teach your child new behaviors. A few examples follow:

Behavior: Children fight over using a bicycle.
Consequence: Removal of bike.

Behavior: Child gets up late for school.
Consequence: Child goes to bed earlier at night.

Behavior: Child splashes others in swimming pool.
Consequence: Child is given time out of the water.

FOUR BASIC RULES

When applying natural consequences, four basic rules we have discussed before need to be observed.

Rule One

Keep your cool. By now you should be familiar with the practice of checking your own emotional state before intervening with your child. You are teaching your child new self-control; therefore, you do not want to model emotionalism. This helps your child to learn to control his or her own energy. It also avoids a major problem that I see quite frequently: when parents are angry or out of control, they frequently administer punishment that is disproportionate to their child's misbehavior. This unfairness causes the child to feel angry, bitter, belittled, and filled with other self-damaging emotions.

Rule Two

This rule goes hand in hand with Rule One. Because it is important I want to draw attention to it.

Speak to your child in a normal tone of voice and be sure to get your child's attention. Do not shout, scream, or raise your voice. Definitely do not demean your child by name-calling (lazy, stupid, etc.), repeating all the problems he or she caused you in the past, or threatening the child with corporal punishment. Stay focused on the most immediate behavior and do not bring up the past.

The best way to do this is to go to where your child is and speak to him or her. If you are shouting across three rooms to get the child's attention, you are already on the verge of losing control.

Rule Three

Empower your child by giving him or her choices. Remember that you are trying to create new learning for your child as quickly as possible. Punishment often produces just the opposite result. Making your child aware of the available choices gives him or her the opportunity to acknowledge old behavior and its inappropriateness. With that awareness, he or she can make a better choice.

Rule Four

Immediately apply natural consequences.

Discussed later are natural consequences for typical problem behaviors. I have chosen the most frequent behaviors I see. My suggestions are written in sand; if you have been successful in the past, and/or wish to experiment with other consequences, I encourage you to do so.

ADDITIONAL PROBLEM BEHAVIORS

Toys, Clothes, and Other Objects Left in the Living Room

When it is time for your child to pick up his toys, give a reminder to do so in the manner described previously. Allow a few seconds to elapse and remind the child a second time. If he does not pick up the toys after two reminders, tell the child that he has reached choice point and explain what the consequence will be.

If the child refuses, pick up the toys. I like to suggest that you put them in a bag and not allow him to play with them for a reasonable period of time. After you do this several times, the child will most likely learn to pick up his toys.

As your child learns the new behavior, provide positive reinforcement through praise and acknowledgment. Here is an example.

Richard was a thirteen-year-old boy who was more creative with avoiding chores than most children I have worked with. He would argue a point until he wore out his opponents. His mother was recovering from an illness while working a demanding job. When she reached home she was worn out and was not able to face a barrage of arguments so she did most of the chores herself, including picking up Richard's clothes in every room of the house.

His mother and I decided it was time for Richard to pick up his clothes, do his homework, and be responsible for various chores each day so his mother would not have to be burdened with this additional work. When Richard came to my office he began to expound on the merits of not doing chores. I let him continue for awhile as he hammered home his points with great conviction and confidence. I told him that if he agreed to pick up his toys and clothes I would make a contract or agreement with him that he would be pleased with. We made an agreement that his mother would not nag him or complain about him. In addition, we added a small incentive for his cooperation.

As we discussed these arrangements, Richard was intransigent—he did not want to change. I knew we would have to apply a negative consequence to increase his motivation. We decided that if he did not pick up his things by a particular time, the other members of the household would throw his clothes, books, homework, games, and other belongings into a large garbage bag hung on the outside of his bedroom door. His brother was especially delighted about this agreement and participated eagerly.

On the following visit, Richard complained that everything was messed up in the bottom of the garbage bag and he thought it was unfair. We briefly discussed the fact that life was sometimes unfair and that he could make decisions to improve his condition. I pointed out that he had the power of choice. If he chose to make poor choices then he had to deal with the consequences. Gradually, as Richard realized that his family and I were united, he began to pick up his things.

Richard never reached 100 percent improvement but he did reasonably well in learning to put his litter away, falling into self-pity on occasions. Many times he surprised me by volunteering to do laundry and help clean house in order to gain some privileges. The net gain by Richard was considerable.

Child Not Dressed and Ready for School on Time

Many children have trouble getting ready for school on time. As a parent you know that it is you who pays the price for this behavior while your child remains unmotivated. I have found good success with the following method, which allows the child to choose whether he wants to be embarrassed.

As time approaches for your child to leave the house, remind him that it is time to get dressed. Give a second reminder and then place the choice in your child's hands so that he knows what the consequence of not being ready on time will be.

If your child is not dressed as the school bus approaches or the car pool shows up, have him continue dressing on the bus or in the car. Make sure the child takes along all the clothes that he needs. An alternative to this is to place socks, shoes, pants—whatever clothing the child does not usually have on—on the front steps when it is time to leave the house.

Some parents feel embarrassed when I suggest this. If they do, I tell them to let the school bus driver, the car pool driver, and the teacher know that they are following the advice of their therapist to help their child. Most parents relax as I point out that they are more likely to be respected for their efforts than chagrined by their children's behavior. As the new behavior is learned, compliment your child on his or her good choice.

Jeshe, who we discussed earlier, had trouble with her grooming. It was not until we made a point chart, a copy of which is reproduced in Chapter 5, that she began to change her behavior. In the beginning she took her time and dallied the early morning hours away. She had a particularly difficult time combing her hair until she learned new grooming habits. When I suggested this method, Jeshe's mother was concerned that Jeshe would never learn to groom herself properly. I reassured her that I trusted the point chart we had made up and that I believed Jeshe would start to change her habits.

After agreeing that Jeshe's clothes (all but her underwear) would be piled in front of the door and that she would have to finish dressing in the car while other children talked about her, we executed the plan. Jeshe was slow the first day and had to lace her shoes and tuck in her clothes in the car on the way to school, but the peer pressure she faced motivated her to get her clothes on before she left the house. For her mother's part, she needed to remind her daughter only twice to get herself fully dressed before the time came to leave for school.

Misbehaving in Public Places

Most parents dread taking their children into public places and having their children misbehave. We dealt with this problem indirectly in Chapter 11, when I discussed temper tantrums.

Clearly define and review with your child what problem behaviors need to be corrected. Make sure your child understands the behavior ahead of time. If you know the environment you will be entering, e.g., a particular store, restaurant, etc., let your child know what the natural consequences will be for misbehaving and the choices he or she will be making.

If you are going to a grocery or department store, you might choose giving your child a time out at a nonstimulating place in the store as the consequence of any misbehavior. For example, you might have the child wait next to the rest room or in the gift wrap section of a department store, or facing the bread display in the grocery store.

If your child continues to act up, take him or her to the car and enforce a time out (ten minutes) while you wait outside the car.

If your child continues to misbehave, then tell your child he or she will be given a time out at home unless the misbehavior stops, and that you will not take him or her with you the next time.

Failure to Go to Bed on Time or Quiet Down for Sleep

As with all these behaviors, remind your child twice in a normal tone of voice and then place the choice in his or her hands. Here are some examples:

> Some children like the bedroom door open and some like it closed in the evening. As the natural consequence of not going to bed on time, tell your child he or she will have to do so with the door in a position opposite that which is preferred. If the child is frightened of having the door closed, then use a night light in his or her room and tell the child you will shut the door for fifteen minutes, after which you will reopen it if he or she behaves.

> Raghu had trouble going to bed on time. He liked to sleep with the door open and the night light on. I told him that if he did not go to bed on time, I would have his mother close the door and turn off the night light. He told me it would not matter. I thought he was showing some bravado, and tried this tactic but it did not work. His mother told me that Raghu had a little ritual he liked to share with her. She would visit him in bed for a few minutes, tuck him in, read a story for a few minutes, and kiss him good night. We decided to give Raghu the choice between going to bed on time or giving up this ritual. Once we put the new plan into action, Raghu had no more trouble going to bed on time. In this case, we removed a positive consequence if he made a bad choice.

Problems in Another Person's Home

If your child behaves poorly when visiting relatives or friends, define and discuss the behavior you want your child to change before you leave home. While you are visiting, if he or she exhibits a misbehavior that you have not anticipated, let your child know at the time that the new behavior is not appropriate. The best natural consequence in this situation is time out.

When visiting, explain to your friends that your child is learning new behaviors and that you may need to give him or her a time out so that the learning process continues uninterrupted.

If your child misbehaves, follow our formula of reminders and choice so that your child has the opportunity to take control of his or her behavior. If your relatives or friends have children that your child misbehaves with, you will need to separate them. Sometimes it is better to have your child take his or her time out in the car, where other children are less apt to be a distraction.

Mealtime Problems

Mealtime problems generally fall into three categories. The first is not eating a meal, the second is fidgeting and squirming, and the third is being disrespectful.

Not Eating

Does your child hardly touch his food, or play with it on the plate with little food entering his mouth? Does your child complain about the food or claim it does not have any taste?

There are several things you can do to help your child:

1. If your child has always been a light eater, place only small portions of food on the plate. Get feedback from other mothers about how much their children eat. Keep portions small.
2. Check your child's medication level. If he has just taken medication he may not have much appetite. If the dosage is wearing off, wait until after mealtime to give the next dose.

Once you have adjusted your child's food portions and checked medication levels, you are ready to help your child learn new eating patterns. Set up some rules ahead of time. If the child does not eat the evening meal, do not allow any snacks for the next twenty-four hours. Continue this for a few days and you should notice an improvement in your child's appetite at mealtime.

As eating habits improve, introduce snacks as a reward for eating appropriately. If your child falls back into the old pattern, do not allow snacks until improvement is observed.

Explain the rules ahead of time and give your child a specific amount of time to complete the meal. This can vary depending on age. If you select twenty minutes, give a reminder after ten minutes, a second reminder after fifteen minutes, and the choice to eat or leave the table at twenty minutes. If the child starts to eat, allow time to finish. Compliment your child on the good choice and let him or her know snacks will be available tomorrow. Remember to keep your cool.

If for any reason your child continues to be reluctant to eat and you believe weight loss is a problem, discuss this with your pediatrician.

Playing at the Table

If your child has trouble sitting still and is seven years old or younger, break the half-hour mealtime into smaller time segments of ten or fifteen minutes. Let your child practice self-control for shorter periods of time. Allow a reward to be earned for each ten-minute segment. Two points could be redeemed for a reward of his or her choosing. See Chapter 5, "Charting the Course to a New Life: Motivating Your Child to Change His or Her Behavior," for reward ideas. Note that in this instance we are not using natural consequences. If your child is very young you may have to break the time segments into smaller increments of five to seven minutes.

Being Disrespectful and/or Disturbing Others at the Table

If your child acts up at the table and disturbs the family during mealtime it is important to change this behavior for the benefit of everyone concerned. First, carefully describe to your child the behavior you want him or her to change. Let us say your child interrupts you, makes fun of the food, and tries to get siblings to misbehave at the table.

Since there is a variety of misbehaviors that the child can combine and change, give one warning and a choice. Remember to keep your cool. This is especially important because your own emotional reaction can be the stimulation that triggers the very behavior you want to change.

If, after one warning, the child does not make the correct choice, have your child get up from the table and take his or her plate of food to a place away from the table to finish the meal alone. Determine where the child shall go ahead of time. If he or she is sent from the table, do not show any special attention. Simply continue your meal calmly with the rest of the family.

Problems When Traveling

When you travel, make sure that your child is taking medication according to schedule. Boredom will rear its head and it is especially difficult for an ADD child to manage hours of sitting in the car as a passenger. This being the case, your child may seek stimulation at your expense and that usually means that he or she will indulge in provocative behavior to get your attention.

Be sure to bring along as many stimulating toys, playthings, books, etc., as possible. Remember that in your child's mind the present moment of boredom or restlessness is going to last forever. So do not count on your child to respond to threats or rewards that will not be delivered until the end of the trip.

Give the child information about the trip rather than general statements about the length. Break the trip into sections. For example, you might tell him or her, "The first section only takes one-and-one-half hours, and we are half way through that." After the first section, take a break and let the child move around to burn off some energy. Continue this throughout the trip. If the child misbehaves, remove toys and playthings and have him or her sit in the back of the car. Tell your child that he or she must stay there until choosing to behave.

When the child says he or she feels ready to behave, wait another five minutes and then return the toys and let the child return to a preferred position in the car. When traveling with two or more children who are misbehaving, separate them so that they do not compound one another's negative behavior.

If problems continue, pull off to the side of the road. Let the adults and children who have behaved well rest and walk around the car. The misbehaving child must remain in the car. Let the child know that his or her behavior is dangerous and fatiguing to the driver. Tell the child that the trip will now take fifteen or twenty minutes longer. When the child is ready to exhibit self-control start the trip again and return all toys. If he or she acts up again, repeat the same procedure.

It is important to do this without becoming excited or upset. Give your child warnings and choices. Make certain neither the other children nor you denigrate the child for slowing down the trip.

Over the years, I have found that it is extremely important to make sure children take their medication prior to taking a trip. Equally important is to ask children what toys they would like to bring along to occupy them. Then use your own discretion and select additional playthings to ensure that the child will be well occupied for the duration of the trip. Many parents find that working on homework assignments during the first part of the trip, and sometimes offering a reward for work completed, works very well.

Problem Behaviors in General

The previously mentioned behaviors have a common theme: they do not follow a set pattern. They also are not serious behavior problems but are simply troubling or aggravating to the household.

When confronted with situations such as these, you may find it necessary to add the time-out chair to the above natural consequences if the natural consequences are not strong enough motivation to change your child's behavior. This, of course, does not apply to driving in the car, though you can replace this by pulling off the highway when possible and letting the others stretch and walk around while the misbehaving child stays in the car.

Keep in mind that we always want to teach new behavior with the simplest approach. If that does not work, then we need to create more motivation.

Your part is very important, and if you can remain calm, your child will benefit enormously. Remember:

1. It is easier for the child to see that you dislike the behavior and not him or her.
2. Your calmness and rational approach gives the child a chance to match your energy.
3. Your calmness slows the child down so that he or she has a chance to reflect on choices rather than act impulsively.

4. Your calmness removes much of the stimulation the child receives from interacting with you. It decreases his or her motivation.
5. Your calmness suggests that the child has the power to change, encourages him or her to change, and respects the child as an individual.
6. Your calmness redefines the episode as one of learning new skills.
7. Your calmness prevents you from saying things that are demeaning and hurtful to your child.
8. Your calmness helps you to be just and fair in setting up positive and negative reinforcement.

That is quite a remarkable list of gains to be had by simply monitoring your emotions and dealing with each issue as a problem to be solved.

I have not listed all the types of behaviors that might be improved by applying natural consequences. However, I hope I have given enough examples so that you can follow the guidelines above and set up your own consequences for the various behaviors that you want to change.

After experimenting with this list for awhile you may find that setting up a point chart works better for you in certain instances. In that case, follow the instructions given in the chapters dealing with aggression, tantrums, and disrespect.

Remember not to take on too many issues at one time. I do not like to take on more than one issue unless I feel the child can handle it. Be very careful to work on changing one behavior before moving onto the next. If you are working with the simpler behaviors previously listed, you may find that working on two at a time works for you. If, however, you are working on any of the serious behaviors, it is a good idea to get them under control first.

You may find that you can work on disrespect as a serious issue and still teach your child to clean his or her room or go to bed on time. But be careful not to overload your child and yourself.

Earlier we stated that all behaviors are learned and can, therefore, be unlearned. But keep in mind that behavior that has taken years and years to form, that has become a deep habit supported by the nervous system, will take time to change. Be patient. Expect improvement, not perfection. Your child will most likely demonstrate many different ADD traits as he or she grows and will continue to struggle with them even as an adult.

Your child's self-esteem and sense of well-being are at stake. You are helping him to build confidence, accept responsibility, learn new skills, and experience himself as a competent person.

Keep your goals modest, compliment your child for changes, and continue to teach. This is the game of the tortoise and the hare—and the tortoise wins!

GOING FORWARD

This chapter concludes Part II of this book. The material presented in this section works best with children between the ages of four and about fourteen. By the time your child is a teenager your influence starts to wane. This is a natural process as peers begin to have more influence. Your child is also beginning to establish some intellectual independence from you. This increased independence and his larger physical size can make it much more difficult to deal with your child.

Parents of teenagers need to learn to discuss problems, develop compromises, and solve issues cooperatively. The issues that the teenager faces are more serious than the issues of younger children. They have the ability to run away, stay with friends, marry early, become pregnant, and so forth. Your role evolves toward one of guidance and stewardship. We will explore the concerns of adolescents and young adults with ADD at length in Part III.

PART III:
PROBLEMS OF ADOLESCENTS
AND YOUNG ADULTS

Chapter 18

The Challenging Teen Years

Even if teenage children aren't making a sound, it's quieter when they're gone. They put a boiling in the air around them. No wonder poltergeists infest only houses with adolescent children.

John Steinbeck
The Winter of Our Discontent

The primary job of teenagers is to prepare themselves for adulthood and independent living. This transition from childhood to adulthood is a complex process that takes the average child six to eight years to accomplish. Many children, following a normal course of development, will begin this transition around the age of twelve or thirteen and not complete it until their early twenties.

This transition is accomplished in many phases, some of which are beyond the scope of this book. What is relevant here is that in the teen years, the child is expected to develop more and more autonomy and a greater sense of responsibility. He will also begin to develop a new identity in which he begins to see himself as an adult; the teen will experiment with relationships and become more independent in thought.

As the teen's parent, you are intimately involved in this process, which is best described as "letting go." The skills to guide your child through the teen years include discussion, brainstorming, negotiation, and stewardship.

Certainly an important focus of this book has been to develop these guidance skills while teaching the young child to be cooperative. If you started working with your child at an early age you will find you have a head start as your child grows older.

If you are the parent of an adolescent and you are just becoming aware that your child has ADD, the job may be more difficult since a foundation of cooperation may not yet be established.

The ADD teenager faces different challenges from those of younger siblings. As independence increases, the result of making poor choices carries with it greater consequences. The life of an ADD teen is fraught with danger: unwanted pregnancies, drug abuse, severe acting out, theft, and collision with the law, to name a few.

The teen who enters these years feeling unloved and unfairly judged by his family, who has given up trying to study because he believes something is wrong with him, and who is angry with his parents and those in authority generally lacks the self-esteem needed to make good choices.

This book establishes sound guidelines to help you, the parent, guide your ADD teen through these challenging years. Unless you have good rapport with your youngster, most likely you will benefit greatly from working with a therapist knowledgeable about ADD. You may also need to have your child diagnosed and treated in therapy before the techniques suggested in this book will be helpful. The following is an example of how this might work.

CASE EXAMPLES

Cassie

Cassie was fourteen when she came to see me. As she sat in my office, she refused to talk to her mother, told her mother to shut up whenever her mother spoke to her, and was extremely angry. She was failing her first year of high school, and her belligerent attitude was causing such serious problems that her physical safety at school was threatened.

Cassie was clearly in control and her mother felt helpless. At home her mood swings were wild. She would lose her temper for no apparent reason. She frequently cursed at her mother and occasionally struck her. She would not allow her mother to answer the telephone or talk to friends unless it suited her. Her behavior was making life extremely difficult for herself and her family.

Cassie was miserable and did not like herself. Part of her problem seemed to focus on her status as a diabetic and the need to give herself insulin injections.

These problems only touched the surface of an array of family problems that created enormous tension among Cassie, her younger brother, and her mother.

I realized that I was unlikely to be able to help Cassie until she was placed on medication for ADD. Appropriate medication could help her gain some control over her behavior. I spent the session telling her how I felt as an unloved teenager, asking her if she had any similar experiences. We established enough of a connection that she was willing to come back for another visit.

Cassie was not only an ADD child but she suffered from depression as well. However, once medication was introduced she began to show improvement and was able to control herself with effort.

It took several sessions to build her trust in me. I would ask her to draw a picture of her experiences during the week and then discuss them with me. This allowed us to begin to communicate. Gradually, I was able to draw her into a discussion of some of the problems that needed attention.

Over the course of several months Cassie made many changes. I wanted to work on one issue at a time, thus giving Cassie the confidence that she would be able to work with her mother and me to resolve the problems she faced.

First, Cassie's school regime was changed to a home-study program; she soon began to take responsibility for completing her assignments and turn in all her work when due. As a result, her grades have improved. Next, we worked out a fair system for using the telephone. Finally, after several months, we began to work on her verbal tirades. She shared with me that she would feel bad after losing control and was ready to consider trying some measures to contain herself. She made steady progress in this area and we are now working on less damaging ways to express her anger with herself and those around her.

Along the way, we had some serious setbacks when she refused to take her medication. I expected to encounter problems and had contingency plans to manage these challenges as they arose.

As the real Cassie emerged, I found her to be a pleasant youngster who captured my heart. Now she enters my outer office and jokes with the staff. They enjoy seeing her. She is a nice young woman and is beginning to feel much better about herself.

The point of this story is that children such as Cassie have special needs. They are subjected to severe judgments and criticisms by the outside world. They carry this pain behind a protective shield; from that hiding place they strike out. If Cassie had been a few years older and more independent, it might have been too late to reach her. The next vignette discusses just such a case.

Ron

Ron was an executive for a technology company. He came to see me for help with the problems he was facing in going through a divorce. In the process of developing a diagnosis, I found that Ron had ADD and treated him for that as well. We met at regular intervals for several months and he began to deal with his problems more effectively. At one point he mentioned that his oldest son, a senior in high school, was having adjustment problems. As I questioned him further, I found that his son had an extensive history of emotional and behavioral problems. Some of his son's behavior was quite serious. He was chronically truant, hated school, was extremely belligerent, resisted authority, was abusing street drugs, and was well beyond his parents' control.

Ron was convinced that his son, Ron Jr., had ADD and that I could help him. I also thought his son might have ADD, but could not make a clinical evaluation until I saw him. I also questioned whether his son would be willing to consider treatment. I told Ron I could never assist anyone with ADD who was unwilling to participate in counseling.

Ron insisted that he bring his son in for treatment. I doubted his son would come with him, but one day Ron surprised me with the news that the two of them would be coming to see me. Ron Jr. was told by his father that it would be beneficial to his (Ron Sr.'s) therapy for him to meet me.

I was concerned because Ron was not being quite honest with Ron Jr. about his reason for scheduling a visit. I told Ron that he was welcome to bring his son, but that I would be focusing on how he related to the boy and, hopefully, help him build better communication skills. If his son was uninterested in treatment, at least I could coach Ron about avoiding some of the communication pitfalls so many parents of ADD children fall into. Ron agreed to settle for the more modest goals that might not necessarily include his son's participation.

As we started the session, Ron Jr. sat with his arms folded across his chest and said that all therapy was a bunch of crap and he could not remember why he agreed to come in the first place. He said he did not believe his father was being helped and that this session was a waste of time for both of them.

I told Ron Jr. that I agreed that therapy was a waste of time if someone did not believe in it but that I also believed it could be quite valuable for those people who wanted to find a way to help themselves. He said he disagreed with me and thought it was a total waste of time for everyone. While I respected his right to have a different opinion, I was curious about the issues he and his father disagreed on.

The young man explained that he wanted to try home study, but his father insisted that he attend school. At this point I sat back as Ron began to tell his son about the school issue.

Ron began lecturing about the advantages of completing school in a normal high school environment. As he expressed his reasoning his son became more and more agitated. Finally the boy interrupted, insisting that he hated school and refusing to continue. An argument ensued.

I stepped in and said that I did not agree with Ron. I pointed out that it was obvious that his son was unable to continue on the school path that had been chosen by his parents. Some education alternatives needed to be considered.

The session continued in this manner. Near the end, I told Ron I wanted to discuss some of the reasons he and his son were having trouble communicating. I focused on Ron's communication problems.

The biggest problem was that Ron had his own agenda for his son, one that did not take into account the youngster's needs and interests. As a result, Ron was not really listening to his son. The truth was he had not come to terms with the boy's ADD.

Ron continued to alienate his son. They fell into the common trap of the lecturing parent and the bored and angry child. Ron's son felt agitated by being talked down to, and this pattern had probably been repeated weekly for eight or ten years.

At eighteen, Ron's son had the power to make his own choices; after many years of unsuccessful attempts to please his parents, he had given up seeking their approval. Now he sought nurturance in ways that society did not accept. This further alienated him from the help that might otherwise have been available to him from his parents through therapy or through other traditional means. In spite of his good intentions, Ron continued to communicate with his son in ways that only served to drive a greater wedge between them.

This story demonstrates the problems parents of ADD teenagers have when they seek treatment too late. If the teen is abusing drugs, has too much control over his or her parents, is simply too independent, or does not believe in the possibility of improving the situation, he or she is very difficult to help. On the other hand, if the teen shows even a slight interest in getting help, his or her future is filled with promise.

If you suspect that your teenager has ADD, the sooner you can obtain a diagnosis and start treatment, the better chance you have of avoiding the problems Ron encountered.

Chapter 19, "What Parents Need to Know," discusses how to guide your child through the teen years. It offers an overview of the task ahead of you and focuses on building communication skills and developing the art of negotiation. In this and subsequent chapters, we will address most of the teen problems you are likely to encounter.

Chapter 19

What Parents Need to Know

There is nothing more difficult to take in hand, more perilous to conduct, or more uncertain in its success, than to take the lead in the introduction of a new order of things.

Niccolo Machiavelli
The Prince

As you set out to help your ADD teenager, bear in mind that in addition to the challenge of ADD, he or she is going through a major transition toward adulthood. As your teenager sets a course, your role is one of assistance and guidance in facing the major challenges of life. Your task is one of stewardship, providing direction, correcting errors, looking ahead for problems, and infusing your child with self-confidence. You will be helping your teen to manage his or her own life so that he or she can take charge of life in ways that will be constructive and satisfying.

One of the most important skills you need for this challenge is effective communication. Learn how to be fair and work out compromises that encourage your teen's development. Find a way to manage your own frustrations so that they do not interfere with the job at hand. And, most important, let your child know that you care about him or her.

This sounds like a big task, and it is. But there are guidelines that can make the work much easier than it appears.

Take time to examine your own parenting style. How do you manage your teenager? What parenting method do you use? Of the four basic parenting styles outlined as follows, most parents will use one primary method, while borrowing some ideas from other styles. You will see that the first three types of parenting methods fall short for a variety of reasons.

PARENTING STYLES

Neglectful Parents

Neglectful parents do not know how to emotionally support their children. Neglectful parents generally have trouble taking care of themselves. Sometimes they have their own emotional problems. Addiction to drugs may be a factor or personal problems just make parenting too tough for them. Children are an intrusion on these parents because their own lives are unmanageable. These teens are usually left to fend for themselves. They generally feel their parents do not care about them. Feeling unwanted or being in the way is a serious blow to the teen's self-esteem.

Laissez Faire or Lenient Parents

These parents believe that their children will grow up successfully with minimal parental interference. They do not like to set rules or establish limits because they have trouble accepting limits themselves. Their children tend to feel insecure because they lack the structure the parent might provide. ADD children, in particular, need structure because they have difficulty internalizing structure for themselves. These children generally control family dynamics and have difficulty, like their parents, in abiding by society's rules.

Dominating Parents

Dominating parents are overcontrolling parents. Frequently, these parents also had dominating parents. When I was young, I was told that "Children should be seen and not heard at the dinner table." In one sense, these rules tend to get handed down from one generation to the next and sometimes stem from a patriarchal European heritage that goes back several generations. These parents have been unable to change with the times and are generally inflexible. "Don't question me," and "Do as I say or there will be serious consequences," are frequent parental utterances. These parents consider unwavering obedience a virtue. They have little ability to engage their children at a personal level or show support for their children, both of which are particularly important for ADD kids. This parenting style robs children of a sense that they are capable of managing their own problems. Frequently, these children are overprotected, which causes a lack of self-confidence. At times, the combination of anger and rebelliousness within the children causes them to act out. Power struggles ensue. Since some of these children only respect absolute power, they continually bid to obtain it over their parents.

Firm and Loving Parents

These parents follow the types of procedures we outlined earlier in this book. They encourage their children to participate in the decision-making process. They help their children learn from the opportunity to make choices. These parents set limits so that each person in the family is respected and children are protected from harming themselves. They provide the love and acceptance that is so important for ADD children. They are flexible and, whenever possible, try to negotiate agreements. Firm and loving parents understand that ADD teens, like their younger counterparts, more willingly accept decisions and rules if they are encouraged to participate in making them.

As you examine your parenting style, try to look at how your methods helped or hindered your child's progress. Most of us adopt and then modify the style of parenting we inherited from our parents. It is important to reexamine yourself so that you can make the adjustments you need to be an effective parent.

As I look back on my life, I realize that, in general, I used a firm and loving style of parenting when raising my three children. When stress mounted I dropped back into my parents' authoritarian style. Since my two younger daughters, Beate and Monika, were not troublesome, I acted, for the most part, as a caring parent that set firm guidelines. Manuela, my ADD daughter, was much more of a challenge and I frequently moved into a more controlling and demanding style of parenting with her, which I am certain aggravated her problems rather than lessened them.

I spoke earlier of stewarding or guiding your children through their teen years. A few guidelines can make this task easier for you. Following are some of the pitfalls to avoid.

PARENTAL PITFALLS

Not Focusing on a Solution to a Problem

When your teen has a problem in school, takes the car without asking, breaks curfew, or in some way creates a problem, it is important to focus on solving the problem. This sounds simple enough, but most parents do not do it. They get caught in their own agendas. Most frequently, they become angry and vent their frustration on the teen. Other times they react without thinking and discipline their teenager too severely. Usually they forget that the simplest way to deal with the problem is to define it and work toward a solution. The story of Ron in Chapter 18 indicates how he was too focused on his own agenda to examine his son's school problems and work toward a creative solution, such as considering an alternative type of school or home study. The parent needs to define the problem, make a fair assessment of the teenager's ability to be responsible, and invite the teen to help develop a solution. The focus should be clearly on avoiding the problem in the future while giving the teen as much power as possible in the decision-making process.

Lecturing

Most parents get caught in the trap of lecturing to their child. Lecturing is one-way communication and does not help resolve a problem. Ron's son had heard his father expound upon the merits of attending regular school for many years. The boy's response was to tune out. The lecture was not received; it was pointless. What was worse, it caused his son to become agitated and seek unhealthy ways to release his frustration. Lecturing causes the teen to feel talked down to like a child; it disempowers, erodes his sense of self-esteem, and builds resentment and anger.

The opposite of lecturing is listening. If Ron had listened to his son explain why he hated school, Ron might have gained some valuable information. Information gathering is important so that a realistic assessment can be made. None of that is possible when one is delivering a soliloquy.

Nagging

Has a parent, boss, friend, or significant other ever nagged you? For a moment remember how that made you feel. Did you just want it to end? If it was about a familiar theme, did you just ignore it, letting it roll off your back? How did you feel afterward? You probably felt resentful, angry, and frustrated.

Your teenager feels the same way. Nagging simply does not work for either of you. It may temporarily release your frustration but, in the long run, it weakens your relationship with your child. Fortunately, there are far better ways to achieve your objectives. If you need to tell your teen twenty times to do something, it is time to seek alternatives. In Chapter 7, "Lessons for Parents," you will find a detailed discussion of an alternative to nagging the younger child. The same principles apply to the teen years.

Arguing

Arguing results in battle lines being drawn after which each side attempts to win at the expense of the other. This always sets up a win or lose situation. If you have more power, your child loses. If your child is older, has more independence, and walks off, then you lose. The reality is that in either circumstance, you both lose.

In spite of the fact that arguing never works, most parents of teenagers fall into this trap at one time or another. Sometimes it is simply as a way to vent frustration; however, releasing emotions on each other never serves the primary focus, which is to solve the problem at hand.

Spontaneous Problem Discussions

Unless you are a highly skilled negotiator, do not attempt to make decisions about difficult issues on the spot. Many times your adolescent will catch you off guard with unexpected requests or demands for immediate decisions. Requests to problem solve on a moment's notice under pressure puts you in an unfair position. Sometimes this is unavoidable, but most of the time you can tell your teenager that you need advance notice to handle any requests so that you can be fair and listen to what he or she has to say. This allows both of you the chance to listen to each other and to work out compromises and differences. The key to your success in working with your teen will hinge on your ability to negotiate differences with him or her.

If you can avoid these pitfalls, both your effectiveness as a communicator and your ability to help your teenager will be enhanced.

PARENTAL RESOURCES

At this point, you might be wondering what resources are available to help you be a successful parent. The fact is that you have many resources available to you.

The most important step you can take is to determine whether your teen has ADD or not. The next step is to obtain treatment as well as medication, if recommended. I cannot recount the number of children of all ages I have worked with who come for an initial evaluation because their behavior is out of hand. If ADD medication is prescribed, the difference in their behavior and their ability to work cooperatively frequently improves remarkably.

Assuming you have taken these steps, you then have a number of tools available to you. I am including a short list of these tools below to give you an idea of the resources you have at hand.

Negotiate

The art of negotiation begins with developing good communication skills. Focusing on solutions, resisting the temptations to lecture, argue, or nag, while avoiding getting caught on the spot, will serve you well in building your negotiating skills.

Examining your parenting style and focusing on parenting in a firm and loving manner will give you a framework within which you can operate. Reviewing the parenting styles in this chapter that do not work and becoming aware when you are slipping into the laissez faire or domineering styles that tend to emerge when you are under stress can help to keep you on track.

Negotiation with your teenager involves focusing on a solution to a problem or a behavior that is inappropriate. It requires that you sit down with your teen and define the problem clearly. Next, ask your teen what his or her thoughts are about finding a solution. Listen to what your teen says. Should he or she drift into explanation or excuses, allow some drift but gently direct the teen back to looking for a solution by asking for ideas again. If you are upset by what you hear, such as, "All the kids I hang out with smoke pot," either wait until you can be less emotional or say that you need time to digest this information and suggest continuing the negotiation at a later time.

Tell your teen that you want him or her to listen to the ideas you have. If your teen does not offer any suggestions, screams at you, or tries to engage you in an argument, tell him or her that you really want to work out a combined solution. Add that if he or she is unwilling to cooperate right now, you would rather try this again at a later time. Ask your teen to try to think of some solutions. Let your teen know that if he or she cannot think of any solutions, you will make a few suggestions from which he or she can choose.

If you have had poor communication with your teenager, he or she may suspect that you are going to fall into your domineering role. Your teen may not trust you at this stage, so it is important for you to remain focused on looking for a solution. If negotiation fails a few times, you may want to seek counseling if the problem is serious. Most teens I encounter who have trouble negotiating think they will not get fair treatment so they give up before they try.

Keep Your Perspective

Is the problem important and serious or is it more aggravating and bothersome? Let the little things go. If your teen keeps his or her room a mess, just keep the bedroom door closed. If he or she forgets a chore, or does not remember to turn off the lights at night, let it go. If your teen does not dress the way you like, this is not a major issue to negotiate. Save your energy so that you can focus on the larger issues.

Distinguish Between Noncompliance and Incompetence

If your teenager breaks a major rule or fails a subject in school, you need to take the time to distinguish between incompetence and non-compliance. It just might be that your teen does not have the capacity to do what you are expecting of him or her.

Noncompliance is deliberate defiance, such as breaking a curfew, something that the teen knows is against the rules. But failing to per-form a difficult math problem at school may be a simple matter of taking on, or being forced to take on, something that is beyond his or her capacity. The trouble is that this behavior may look the same in either case, since an ADD child is quite capable of using belligerence to cover up a feeling of inadequacy.

It is not always easy to know the difference between noncompli-ance and incompetence. But it is important not to overreact or jump to the conclusion that the teen is being defiant. Examine your own expectations of him or her. You may want your teen to be an Ivy League scholar but, no matter how you push, the dominant challenge is going to be the teen's struggle with ADD. ADD teenagers are for-getful and seemingly unmotivated if they do not have a deep personal interest in what they are doing. It is much better that you spend your time helping them identify those interests rather than pushing them to do something in which they have no interest.

Look Around the Corner

Try to anticipate problems before they occur. If your teen is think-ing about getting a part-time job and his or her schoolwork is poor, or if you are planning to go out of town for a weekend and you know your teenager wants to have a party at your house, prepare yourself in advance to manage forthcoming activities or problems.

Another aspect of being prepared is to discuss problems he or she is likely to encounter. What challenges will your teen meet when dat-ing? How many of his or her friends experiment with drugs? When your teen is alone after school for many hours, how is his or her time spent? It is important to encourage your teen's self-expression, to share experiences and concerns with you so that you can provide guidance.

Ask your teen whether he or she finds that impulsiveness tends to get him or her into trouble. See how your teen responds. Does he or she goof off in front of the opposite sex to the point of embarrassment? Does your teen make promises that cannot be kept? The key to being prepared to help your teenager is to anticipate problems or challenges he or she is likely to encounter and dialogue about them.

Avoid "I Told You So"

When your teen fails, resist the temptation to say, "I told you so." Have your teen discuss feelings about missing a goal or expectation. Share some stories of your own; tell your teen how you felt in a similar situation. If your teen breaks a rule, do not berate him or her. Remind your teen that he or she has a consequence to pay that will help with learning to make better decisions in the future. Avoid lecturing. Encourage your teen to share feelings. ADD teenagers are sensitive and their reactions to disappointing situations can be more prolonged or deeper than those of their peers. There is no need for you to take on your child's emotions. A simple question asking how you might be of help or support through a difficult experience is sufficient.

Accept Your Teen, Disapprove of the Behavior

This is an underlying principle of all recommendations in this book. Your youngster is more than just behavior. Even though you are guiding this behavior, your teen will make mistakes, test you, get confused and be completely human in every aspect. Try to understand the teenager's world. When you were in high school, were you shy? Did you have trouble making friends? Did you act out or try to get attention in immature ways because you were unsure of yourself? Remember that all of your teen's behavior has a reason or motivation behind it. What is that motivation? The more you can perceive life through your teen's lens and not yours, the more you will be able to offer nurture and support.

Consequences

When establishing guidelines and limits, you need to work out with your teen what consequences will follow for breaking rules. It is never too late to set guidelines and limits; the sooner you take a firm hand the easier it should be. Your teenager is no longer a child. You cannot simply demand compliance, particularly with an ADD teen. He or she will want to know the reason for new rules. You need to provide your teen with sound reasoning. Let the teen know his or her behavior affects other members of the family and the community as well.

Your Weapons Are the Removal and the Awarding of Privileges

When negotiating consequences for inappropriate behavior, ask your teenager for input as to what would be a fair privilege to lose. Your teen may be too harsh. Although this is unlikely, it does happen. Start with small losses of privileges and escalate if necessary. The biggest trap parents fall into is punishing too severely.

I just interviewed a thirteen-year-old boy who had all his privileges removed for acting out severely at school and on the school bus. He was not allowed to be with his friends after school or to talk to them on the telephone. He was not allowed to watch television and was grounded for several weeks. In short, he had no incentive to change. His parents were very reluctant to go back on their word. I encouraged them to award a privilege each time he did not act out in class so that he would have an immediate incentive to change. I also referred him to his physician for a review of his medication because I thought his behavior should be more under his control.

After carefully reviewing his case, we discovered that the boy had become overwhelmed by schoolwork he did not understand. At first, his parents and teachers did not recognize the problem. As his grades began to fall, they pressured him to work harder, which only compounded his problems.

If you find that you are not sure what to do, seek some professional guidance. In the case of this thirteen-year-old boy, since I had worked with the family a year earlier, just one visit allowed us to work out the problem.

Differentiate Between Negotiable and Nonnegotiable Issues

Make a distinction between those issues that are not negotiable and those that are. Eventually, as your teenager grows older and more responsible, nearly every issue should become negotiable.

You need to examine which issues are open to negotiation and which are not. Some nonnegotiable issues may have parts that can be negotiated. An example of this might be that no overnights are allowed during the school week. If, however, a school project is nearing completion and your teen can benefit from working with a friend, you may want to relax this rule so that they can work late together.

A FEW NOTES

These tools can help you guide your teenager through the challenges faced as he or she grows toward adulthood. If you apply them, you can avoid making many mistakes. As parents, we do not have a built-in guidance system that helps us reach our goal. We need to learn from trial and error. I have mentioned frequently that I learn as much from the patients who visit me as they do from me. I learn which interventions work and which do not, and why some succeed and others fail. Mostly, I learn by asking a lot of questions. If I work on a problem issue and my interventions do not yield immediate or expected results, I realize that I need more information. I keep an open mind and continue to gather information.

Do not be too hard on yourself when working with your teenager. The most important thing you can do is focus on solving a problem and enlisting the aid of your youngster. You will learn by trial and error, as I do. I follow these guidelines and it makes my work much easier. If you find that you are following the guidelines and still you remain stuck, I suggest you seek professional assistance.

Take care of yourself. Working with ADD teens can be very demanding. Find ways to let go and relax. Share with your partner if you have one. Take breaks when you need them. Schedule weekends away from the house to renew yourself if you can. Above all, do not expect to be perfect. Join a CHADD (Children and Adults with Attention Deficit Disorder) group and share with other ADDers and their parents.

Get massages, practice yoga, meditate, and get involved in other activities so that you add balance to your life.

In the next chapters, I will be discussing some of the more frequent problems you might encounter with your teenager.

Chapter 20

Adolescent Anger

*What other dungeon so dark as one's own heart! What jailer so
inexorable as one's self.*

Nathanial Hawthorne
The House of the Seven Gables

Many teens with ADD overreact and are hypersensitive to criticism. Frequently, the slightest provocation makes them angry. Most other teens find ways to manage anger without acting out, but research indicates that over 40 percent of the teens diagnosed with ADD have problems with anger control. When an ADDer releases anger in a way that harms others, serious consequences can follow.

Swearing at a parent, threatening a parent or sibling with physical harm, striking someone, or damaging property are serious behavior issues that must be addressed immediately.

If your teen engages in these behaviors, one of the best ways to manage them is to talk to your teenager when he or she is not angry and say that you understand that this anger is real. Tell your teen it is okay to be angry but it is not okay to act out his anger in ways that violate the safety of others. It is extremely important to emphasize that the emotion of anger itself is normal and it is okay to feel it. However, we must learn ways to express it that will not harm others or ourselves. Explore some of the safe, positive ways that your teen might release anger. Set agreements with your teen to release emotions in ways that are neither destructive nor dangerous. Many teens have success releasing their anger in their bedroom with the door shut. Banging on the bed or pillow or screaming into the pillow can provide a good release of pent-up emotions. One young man I worked with hung a punching bag in his room and beat on it when he was angry. He liked this release and enjoyed the fact that it helped him build stronger arm muscles.

You may not be successful in finding ways to help your teenager contain anger, or your teen may not appear to be making much of an effort to do so. Should this be the case, you should seek professional help. Some teenage ADDers have a condition known as conduct disorder. The *Diagnostic and Statistical Manual of Mental Disorders* (DSM-IV), defines conduct disorder (CD) in the following way.

CONDUCT DISORDER

A. A repetitive and persistent pattern of behavior in which the basic rights of others or major age-appropriate societal norms or rules are violated, as manifested by the presence of three (or more) of the following criteria in the past 12 months, with at least one criterion present in the past 6 months:

Aggression Toward People and Animals

(1) often bullies, threatens, or intimidates others
(2) often initiates physical fights
(3) has used a weapon that can cause serious physical harm to others, e.g., bat, brick, broken bottle, knife, or gun
(4) has been physically cruel to people
(5) has been physically cruel to animals
(6) has stolen while confronting a victim
(7) has forced someone into sexual activity

Destruction of Property

(8) has deliberately engaged in fire setting with the intention of causing serious damage
(9) has deliberately destroyed others' property

Deceitfulness or Theft

(10) has broken into someone else's house, building, or car

(11) often lies to obtain goods or favors or to avoid obligations (i.e., "cons" others)

(12) has stolen items of nontrivial value without confronting a victim (e.g., shoplifting without breaking and entering; forgery)

Serious Violations of Rules

(13) often stays out at night despite parental prohibitions, beginning before age 13 years

(14) has run away from home overnight at least twice while living in parental or parental surrogate home (or once without returning for a lengthy period)

(15) often truant from school, beginning before age 13 years

B. The disturbance in behavior causes clinically significant impairment in social, academic, or occupational functioning. (Reprinted with permission from the *Diagnostic and Statistical Manual of Mental Disorders,* Fourth Edition. Copyright 1994 American Psychiatric Association.)

If your ADD teen shows signs of a conduct disorder, you do need help. Should this be the case, I suggest you contact a professional as soon as possible. If money is a problem there are usually low cost or sliding fee county resources that work with these problems. If you do not know where to begin, talk to your doctor or call the local battered women's association for information and guidance.

Some teenagers exhibit a condition that is less serious than conduct disorder known as oppositional defiant disorder (ODD). The criteria for ODD are as follows.

OPPOSITIONAL DEFIANT DISORDER

A. A pattern of negativistic, hostile, and defiant behavior lasting at least six months, during which four (or more) of the following are present:

(1) often loses temper

(2) often argues with adults

(3) often actively defies or refuses to comply with adult's requests or rules
(4) often deliberately annoys people
(5) often blames others for his or her mistakes or misbehavior
(6) is often touchy or easily annoyed by others
(7) is often angry or resentful
(8) is often spiteful or vindictive (Reprinted with permission from the *Diagnostic and Statistical Manual of Mental Disorders,* Fourth Edition. Copyright 1994 American Psychiatric Association.)

Four of the above criteria must prevail for a period of time lasting at least six months and the disturbance in behavior must cause clinically significant impairment in social, academic, or occupational functioning.

To meet the clinical criteria for ODD and CD, a youngster must exhibit these listed behaviors for six months or longer. Many ADDers demonstrate some of the above characteristics but do not meet the rigorousness of six months of consistent behavior. Or they exhibit some symptoms with less intensity, so that their overall ability to function is not impaired.

Approximately 30 to 40 percent of the teenagers I treat have both ADD and one of these two disorders. Conduct disorder occurs less frequently than oppositional defiant disorder, but both are treated as true mental or emotional illnesses. Many parents, not understanding the nature of these disorders or their symptoms, are truly perplexed as to why their children behave as they do. Other parents deny the seriousness of aggressive misbehavior and refuse to deal with it appropriately.

But ODD and CD are cries for help. With good professional attention, most teenagers with ADD do learn better behavior. In a sense, these behaviors are manifestations of the rage felt by a child overwhelmed by ADD. Frustrated and having poor impulse control, the ADD child gives up, acts out, or strikes out.

The suggestions given in the previous chapter can help you to work with your child if he or she has ODD. You may find that you are successful helping your teen, particularly when medication is prescribed and taken. Frequently, ODD is an outgrowth of a child's experiences of unfair treatment at a younger age. Rarely does the teenager see defiance. Rather, in his or her behavior the teen feels he or she is correcting perceived wrongs. In all cases, early intervention is extremely important. If you find that your teen does not respond to your new efforts and understanding, it is important to seek treatment.

PREVENTIVE PARENTING

You can reduce the risks of your teen developing CD or ODD. The following suggestions will help you treat problem behavior before it gets out of control.

Early Identification and Treatment of ADD

If you suspect your teenager has ADD, the sooner you seek a diagnosis from a qualified specialist, the sooner you can help your youngster. Early intervention is the key to helping your teen learn to cope with the special challenges he or she faces.

Medicate As Prescribed

If your child has ADD and medication is recommended, it is very important that you ensure that your child takes medication according to the doctor's specifications.

Understand ADD

Your ADD child will have strengths and limitations. It is important for you to understand his or her limitations and not push your teen beyond capacity. Adjust your expectations accordingly. Most of the problems I have presented in this book have resulted from parents holding too tightly to personal agendas for their children and not taking the time to understand their ADD child's capabilities and shortcomings. In Chapter 1, I shared my own struggle with this problem as a parent. The case study in Chapter 18 about Ron and his son describes another parent's problem in understanding his teenager.

Acknowledge Your Child's Emotions

This may be more difficult. When your teenager is angry or upset, try to acknowledge this emotional state. You do not necessarily have to understand or agree, but you can acknowledge that your teen is experiencing difficulty. No doubt you and your teen will interpret the same experiences through very different perceptual lenses. In fact, there will be times when you will wonder if you are both from the same planet!

Nurture and Support Your Teen

Let your youngster know that you care for him or her, but do not agree with or support inappropriate behavior. If the acting out is directed at you, it may be difficult for you to reach out to your child immediately. This is okay. Once you have had time to work through your emotions, tell your child that you are human and reacted by being upset. Try to resolve the problem. Make it clear to your teen that you make a distinction between the teen and the behavior.

Try to do fun things together. Forgive quickly; let misbehavior go once it has been corrected. Resist the temptation to say, "I told you so."

Be a Firm and Loving Parent

This does not mean that you accept misbehavior but that you guide your child through firmness. Avoid authoritarian parenting as much as possible. Review the parenting styles described in Chapter 19. Check your style from time to time.

Negotiate Issues

Work with your teen to adopt rules and limits that are appropriate. Discuss consequences. Listen, listen, and listen some more to what your teen has to say. If your child is asking for too much responsibility, communicate that you need to set certain limits. Stand firm in your decision but let your teen know that, as he or she grows and demonstrates the ability to handle responsibility, you will be willing to rethink and modify your position.

Some children respond negatively to phrases such as "accepting responsibility" or "being responsible." Too often such phrases are used in a judgmental way that they perceive as an insult. If you find this to be true with your child, look for less annoying ways to express your meaning. For example, use a different approach: "I don't think

I'm ready to let you take that on yet" or "I'd like to see you develop a little more self-control before you take that on."

If your ADD teen knows that you are trying to work with him or her and provide support, you minimize the possibility that he or she will resort to defiance. Because self-expression is encouraged, the acting out is not necessary.

Review the suggestions given in Chapter 19, "What Parents Need to Know."

Chapter 21

School Problems

The Widow Douglas, she took me for her son, and allowed she would sivilize me: but it was rough living for me in the house . . . and when I couldn't stand it no longer, I lit out.

Mark Twain
Adventures of Huckleberry Finn

Children graduating from elementary school to junior high or from junior high to high school frequently need extra guidance to make the changes they will be confronting. The move from a structured environment to a less structured one can be a difficult challenge for ADD teens who tend to have trouble with change in general. New demands and responsibilities can easily cause them to feel overwhelmed.

In addition to managing this stress, the ADD teenager must learn to handle more advanced studies and longer assignments. This means that take-home projects are more frequent, and the need to remember previous lessons in language, math, and the sciences is required.

The youngsters who strained to get their elementary school work completed must now call upon new resources to organize, prioritize, plan, and break assignments into smaller segments. Frequently, these tasks are beyond the ability of many ADD teens and they begin to falter. In my counseling practice I see this happen again and again. Typically, ADD teens will keep their faltering a secret until report cards appear. By that time they are overwhelmed and have given up.

Other ADD children have trouble remembering earlier lessons. What has been learned, or probably only partially learned, is forgotten quickly. Foreign languages, math, and the sciences are extremely difficult for many ADD teens because of their memory problems.

Teachers in high school expect students to be more self-reliant and responsible for obtaining the information they need. Ideally, if ADD teens can tell their teachers that they have ADD and have trouble remembering oral assignments or taking timed tests, help may be available. Many teachers give ADD students special consideration when taking tests, or when managing memory and organizational tasks.

Peer pressure to conform and the fear of being different from friends make it particularly difficult for ADD teens to speak up for themselves. As parents, you will probably be required to advocate for your youngsters to obtain the help they need from their school.

Many ADD teens silently give up and act out, creating behavior disturbances at school and at home. They feel caught between a school system that does not work for them and parents who do not understand their difficulties.

GUIDELINES FOR PARENTS WHOSE TEENAGERS HAVE DIFFICULTY IN SCHOOL

If your teenager has difficulty in school, the following guidelines will be helpful.

Advocacy

If possible, it is a good idea to keep your teenager in a regular high school. To do this, you may need to talk to teachers and the school staff to explain the situation. If you can obtain help from teachers— and you usually can—then your teen can remain in his or her present school and continue regular education.

IEP

You may find it necessary to talk to the school administrators and request the development of a program that is suited to your child's particular needs. The development of an individual educational plan (IEP) is a comprehensive process that involves your child's teachers, the dean, the school principal, the school psychologist, and other specialists as needed. Individual educational plans were discussed in Chapter 14; I suggest you review that information again if you find your teen has special needs that can be served by an individualized study program.

Private Schools

Many private schools work particularly well with ADD children. If you are able to afford private education, the more individualized attention available at many of these schools can help to make your teen's educational experience a positive one.

Alternative High Schools

In California, every county has an alternative high school for children who need more than the traditional classrooms can provide. Classes are small and the teachers are available to assist each child. They check up on the teens, and for the most part, allow the youngsters to progress at their own rate.

Home Study

I have seen many ADD teenagers manage home study well. Assignments are given in abbreviated form and the work is turned in weekly. The child follows the school's curriculum and graduates with his or her regular class. I recommend this approach to parents when other measures fail. Many children who benefit from home study find that after a year or two they are able to return to school. Frequently, they return to their regular class for their final semester of high school.

Cassie (Chapter 18) found she was able to do this. As of this writing she is returning to school following home study for three semesters. Of course, home study means that a parent or adult guardian who is able to supervise the teen's studies must be at home with the child during regular school hours.

Tutors

Tutors are much less expensive than private schools and can tailor their assistance to fit your child's needs. A tutor can be an excellent resource for teaching your child how to study, what to study, and how to organize his or her academic life. Frequently, this kind of individualized assistance can make it possible for your teen to remain in regular high school. Contact your school's counselors for a list of recommended tutors.

Parental Help

In Chapters 14 and 15, I described a number of checklists and interventions that can be useful when working with elementary school students. Many of these checklists can be easily adapted to the needs of your high school teen. They will help you to uncover valuable information about your teenager's specific weaknesses, and provide suggestions to help improve study skills. I encourage you to reread those chapters. A quick review follows.

TYPICAL PROBLEMS

Forgets Books

Either have your teen bring home all schoolbooks every night or, if possible, buy a second set of books to keep at home.

Unclear About Assignments

Have your teen write down each assignment during class time and ask the teacher to check it for accuracy and misinformation.

Forgets, Works Too Fast,
Insists No Homework Was Assigned

Set aside one hour each day to have your teen do an assignment of your choice. If after several days he or she still forgets, increase the time to ninety minutes until he or she brings classroom assignments home.

Refuses to Study

Revoke privileges. Privileges are earned after homework is completed.

Clarifying Responsibilities

Do not fall into the pattern of completing assignments for your ADD teen or asking siblings to complete them. This is not the parents' responsibility and it is a waste of time for all those involved.

As a parent you should:

1. Help your teen set up a regular time for doing homework every day.
2. See that your teen starts and finishes studying at the agreed-upon time. Remove privileges if assignments are not completed.
3. Keep the family out of the study area.
4. Help your teen get started if he or she has trouble starting or breaking down a long assignment into smaller sections. Do not do the work for your child.
5. If possible, help explain problems or assignments he or she does not understand.
6. Ask to see the completed assignment and make sure your teen places it with his or her books to ensure that your child remembers to take it to school the next day.

Your ADD teenager will probably require some parental assistance to manage the challenges of high school. Many parents become bogged down with their teen's school problems and find themselves frustrated or feeling hopeless. But, as previously mentioned, it is important to keep a broad perspective.

During their children's teen years many parents find themselves facing the reality that their offspring may not be successful academically. They fear their children's future welfare is in jeopardy without a first-class education and good college choices. These fears tend to cause parents to push their ADD children beyond their capacity, potentially creating a great deal of turmoil. Frequently, this undermines teens' self-confidence, which for most ADDers needs a boost in the first place. I believe it is more important to find ways to build your child's self-esteem and self-confidence than to expect academic excellence.

I have found that ADD teens who feel good about themselves and understand their weaknesses and strengths negotiate the challenges of adult life well. These qualities are more important to the young adult than an education at a good college. Many ADD children mature a bit later in their years than their non-ADD counterparts. Many ADD teens go on to a junior college that allows them more time to complete course work. Others find increased motivation at a later age which, when combined with improved study skills, allows them to achieve a higher education. Many others develop good careers in sales, contracting, various types of entrepreneurship, or other niches that showcase their creativeness and abilities.

In my own history, I barely made it through high school. I honestly do not remember taking any books home or doing homework. When I graduated from high school I looked at my life opportunities and became frightened. I decided I would find some way to attend junior college. It took me three years to complete two years of work. I built strong study skills and my fear motivated me to succeed. I transferred to the University of California and called upon all my learning resources and study aids and graduated with decent grades.

I used my other talents to develop a career as a stockbroker. When I left the business world after twenty years of success, I felt so good about myself that the challenge of graduate school did not seem that frightening. To me, it became another challenge, not any different from the obstacles I had conquered in the past. The confidence I felt as an adult in changing careers at midlife was probably a hundred times greater than I experienced as an eighteen-year-old.

The point of my personal story is that it is helpful to keep a wide perspective on education. I felt inferior at school, and many of my friends were much better students than I was. At that time I did not like to think about my future because I thought my prospects were limited.

The way I had thought about myself brought up feelings of inadequacy because of the unfair comparisons I made. My brother was very intelligent and scholarly, and I lived with this knowledge every day. I had no idea that I might mature and view life differently, or that I might be creative in finding life pursuits that fit my temperament and nature, or that I might get excited about a career, and throw myself into it.

Academic education is important, but it is also important not to let parental anxieties obscure the larger picture that a teen can have a promising life whether or not he or she is a top student.

Chapter 22

Winning with Drug and Alcohol Problems

I recun a body that ups and tells the truth when he is in a tight place, is taking many considerable resks, though I ain't had no experience, and can't say for certain. . . . Well, I says to myself, at last, I'm going to chance it! I'll up and tell the truth this time, Though it does seem most like setting down on a keg of powder and touching it off.

Mark Twain
Adventures of Huckleberry Finn

Regardless of economic backgrounds, many young people experiment with drugs and alcohol during their teen years. A recent report issued by the U.S. Department of Education indicated that 89 percent of high school seniors have used alcohol and 24 percent have used marijuana. Two-thirds of teens report that they have been drunk at least once. Even more startling is the fact that 75 percent of eighth graders have had at least one drink of alcohol.

The thought of teenagers using drugs and alcohol is frightening to parents. Yet alcohol and marijuana experimentation by teenagers, for better or for worse, is considered a relatively normal part of their developmental experience. Many teens believe they can experiment with drugs behind their parents' backs. They are correct! Although more and more parents are becoming aware of this problem, disbelief and denial cause them to miss many of the telltale signs of drug usage.

Most adolescents drink or smoke pot only occasionally. Others experiment with these substances and find that drugs are not for them. Still others will use them only to be sociable—for example, at parties. Reliable statistics are hard to come by, but probably about 15 percent of teens will develop drug problems and fewer than that will become addicted or dependent on drugs.

Drug use escalates over a period of time, so parents who are aware of the signs have an excellent chance of catching a problem while it is still developing. Most experts agree that teens use marijuana as a launching pad to abuse heavier drugs such as cocaine and speed (methamphetamines). I believe that children who "graduate" to heavier drugs are the ones who do not feel good about themselves. They find an escape through drugs, as well as the support of other dropouts with whom they identify. These temptations are extremely compelling for those youngsters who have not been able to find more constructive paths of acceptance.

ADD teens are in a high-risk group for alcohol and drug use because of the rejection they experience from peers, family members, society, and their own negative self-judgment. Furthermore, their impulsiveness and need for instant gratification, particularly when they find little gratification elsewhere, make it difficult for them to resist medicating themselves on the street corner.

Contrary to what some people believe, the use of medicine to treat ADD reduces the likelihood of teens succumbing to "self-treatment" on the street. Medicine helps reduce the frustration and pain ADD children experience, and gives them more control over their nervous systems so that they can make better decisions and feel better about themselves.

ADD TEENS AND SUBSTANCE ABUSE

Toward a State of Self-Esteem, * the report issued in 1990 by a California task force, indicated a definite connection between substance abuse and self-concept:

> Research does solidly document a connection between substance abuse and self-concept, a broader notion which includes self-esteem. Psychological theory suggests that a failure to develop a healthy concept of one's self, either early in childhood or in later relationships with parents, can create a condition ripe for drug and alcohol abuse.

Toward a State of Self-Esteem. (January, 1990). The final report of the California task force to promote self-esteem and personal and social responsibility. California Department of Education, P.O. Box 944272, Sacramento, CA 94244-2720.

At least one major study concluded that low levels of self-esteem are the cause, not the result, of deviant behavior. In other words, alcoholic or drug addicts behave as they do because of low self-esteem, rather than developing low self-esteem as the result of deviant behavior. (p. 88)

The authors conclude, "The prevention and treatment of alcohol and drug abuse should focus on the development of a healthy sense of self . . . that is of sustaining self-esteem through the normal problems of living, accompanied by a parallel development in related personal values and choices of drug-free social involvements" (p. 90).

The focus of this book has been to help you understand your ADD child and learn how to show that you respect and value him or her. I mentioned earlier in the book that children complete school and then face life with the skills and mind-set they have developed over the first sixteen or eighteen years living with their parents. This is why I believe that building your child's self-esteem and helping develop the behavioral skills needed to function successfully should be your top priority.

ADD teens have a higher incidence of drug and alcohol abuse than their peers do. Their struggles, both within themselves and with society, tend to leave them feeling negatively about themselves. An eight-year study by Dr. Russell Barkley found that children with ADD and conduct disorder were more apt to abuse drugs or alcohol than children who had only ADD. This suggests that ADD alone does not necessarily predict future substance abuse, but it definitely indicates that parents must be alert to the fact that ADD children are at risk. If your child has ADD combined with oppositional defiant disorder or conduct disorder you must to be particularly alert to signs of drug use.

SIGNS OF DRUG USE

Parents need to educate themselves about signs of drug use by their children. Usually a number of tangible and behavioral signs indicate that teenagers are using drugs.

Hypodermic needles, vials, white powder, and marijuana leaves are certain evidence of drug usage. Teens are sometimes careless and leave pipes, pills, butts, seeds, and other drug paraphernalia in their rooms. If you find any of these articles, you have "hard" evidence that your child is using drugs. The sweet odor of marijuana on a teen's clothes is a sure giveaway that he or she has been smoking pot.

Some teens will burn incense or use other scents to cover up the smell of drugs. If your teenager starts using incense or similar scents in his or her room you should be watchful. There are also other indicators that your child is probably using alcohol or drugs. The following are "soft" signs that may point to the use of drugs by your teenager.

Physical Deterioration

If your teen becomes less concerned with appearance, becomes indifferent to hygiene and grooming, or changes the way he or she dresses, this might indicate the use of drugs. If physical appearance changes, eyes are bloodshot, or pupils are dilated, you may be seeing another warning sign. If your youngster seems less sharp, speaks slower, or has more trouble remembering, the change in behavior may also be a warning sign. If you notice an increase in laziness or a loss of energy and the teen appears less interested in the activities he or she formerly enjoyed, this behavior could be drug related.

School Performance

If your child has a marked downturn in school grades, or studies less, or does not complete assignments that are usually completed, these are soft signs that he or she might be using drugs.

Behavior Change

If your teen changes friends or the group of people he or she has socialized with, or is uneasy talking to you about new friends, your teen could be using drugs. If the child is more hostile or irritable, becomes upset when you ask about activities, or how he or she spends free time, you may have cause for concern. If your teen shows a diminished interest in activities, hobbies, and sports, this could be an indication of substance abuse. Should you find large amounts of money in your teen's pockets, if he or she has trouble with the police, or if you catch your child stealing or shoplifting, he or she may be dealing in drugs or breaking the law to get money for drugs.

If your teen redecorates his or her room and you find drug-related posters, magazines, or slogans, chances are the child is beginning to identify with drug culture. A collection of beer cans may be age appropriate or it may be a signal that your teen is having trouble with alcohol.

Most important, if your teen shows hostility when you talk to him or her about drugs, chances are high that he or she is concealing information from you.

Some of these signs may not be specifically drug related. They could indicate that your teen is experiencing trouble at school, a drop in self-esteem, an increase in ADD difficulties, a depressive episode, or other problems that are not drug related. If the soft signs are combined with any evidence of drug paraphernalia, or you find a number of the behavior changes just discussed, you definitely need to further investigate the possibility of drug use by your youngster.

MANAGING DRUG USE

If some of the above signs are familiar and you believe your teenager may be using drugs, be forthright and ask directly in a calm, nonaccusatory tone. Listen to how your child responds. Look for signs of deception, embarrassment, prepared responses, blushing, stammering, or any other indication that he or she is hiding something.

Many teenagers will go to great lengths to deceive you about their use of drugs. They may deny using drugs in spite of concrete evidence to the contrary. If your teen takes this position, do not get into a prolonged fight or argument. Never confront your youngster when he or she is high or drunk. If you hear such common responses as, "I only tried it once," "That stuff is not mine," "I was tricked into trying it," or "Everyone does it," you know your teen has a problem. If you actually catch your youngster high or drunk it is entirely possible that it is not his or her first time; in the past, the child may have just slipped past you, stayed overnight at a friend's house, or snuck home late when you were asleep to avoid being discovered.

If possible, try to assess the seriousness of your teen's usage. If he or she drank too much on a Saturday night at a party and does this rarely, or if he or she was celebrating a school athletic victory, or acknowledges having three or four beers on a weekend night, your teen is probably engaging in what these days is age-appropriate behavior. Keep an eye on this behavior, but do not panic.

Check with friends and neighbors who have teens to obtain more information and a greater perspective on how the average teenager socializes. Whatever your findings, good or bad, you need to set time aside to talk to your teen about the use of alcohol or drugs. If he or she is drinking socially, it is important to formulate some basic rules to minimize the inherent risks.

Typical rules are as follows.

1. Never drink and drive.
2. Do not ride in a car with a driver who has been drinking.
3. If a party gets wild, leave.
4. Designate a driver who will stay completely sober.

Many parents tell their teen to call home for a ride or give him or her cab money to get home to help their teen abide by the rules.

If you believe or suspect that your youngster has a problem with drugs, seek professional help. Most counties have substance abuse treatment centers where you can make an appointment for a consultation. Any therapist who works with teenagers can provide you with help as well. Do not minimize drug problems or fall into denial about your child's activity. Your denial only compounds the problem.

Keep in mind that your goal is to prevent your child from becoming an addict or an alcoholic and from using drugs to escape problems. Teenagers are highly susceptible to peer influences that may glamorize the use of alcohol and drugs. The earlier you confront and deal with these issues appropriately, the less chance your child has of abusing or becoming dependent on drugs.

A FINAL NOTE

If your child is using drugs or you simply need to talk to him or her about this subject, reread the suggestions given in Chapter 19 on communicating with your teenager. Even if you are shocked by what you discover, do not discard the suggestions given for improving your relationship with your teenager. As you discuss this issue, you need to listen to your teen. You may find that he or she has a lot of information to share with you about what his or her social set is doing. If your teen feels you are really listening, he or she may be secretly pleased that this issue has surfaced, particularly if previously ill at ease with it, which is the case with many teenagers. Your teen may be concerned and not know what steps to take or how to handle the pressure to "party" with friends. The child may also be frightened that you have found out and be concerned about what punitive action you might be considering. You simply have no way of knowing how your teen will react. Many parents fear the abuse of drugs by their ADD teen more than most challenges their teen brings to them. Do not let your fears prevent you from dealing with this critical problem in a patient, firm, but understanding way.

Parents who discover their teenager is using drugs need to remind themselves that they disapprove of their child's actions and not the child. This is extremely important. Drug use, if it occurs, is another challenge that you and your teen must face together and should be dealt with from a rational, problem-solving viewpoint. Remember, the earlier you confront and deal directly with this issue, the better chance your teen has of avoiding addiction or having to go through a recovery program. Your job is to focus on finding a solution and changing the troublesome behavior.

Remember that drug and alcohol use only gets worse with time. If your teenager begins to use drugs or alcohol you will most likely receive "soft" signs that he or she is doing so. The earlier you discuss the consumption of drugs, the sooner you can take corrective action. As the parent of an ADD child, particularly if your teen has been acting out, or displaying the symptoms of a conduct or oppositional defiant disorder, you need to intervene early. If your efforts to obtain information do not yield results, or if your teen disregards the limits you set regarding drug and alcohol abuse, you need to obtain professional help.

Chapter 23

Additional Teenage Problems

I can't go on . . .
I really
can't go on
I swear
I can't go on
so
I guess
I'll get up
and go on

Dory Previn

There are a number of behaviors you will need to deal with as your teenager continues development toward adulthood. The issues that will arise are typical of the challenges most parents solve with their teenagers. If you are just starting to work with the particular challenges of your child's ADD, or you have been having difficulty dealing with each issue as it occurs, guidance on the following issues should be helpful.

MESSY ROOMS

With few exceptions, this is a problem parents may have to own and deal with themselves. Your youngster's room is private territory. My advice is to close the door so you do not have to see the mess. ADD teen rooms probably are messier than most teen rooms, but no researcher has deemed it important enough to conduct a study. In spite of my advice on this issue, many parents still have trouble letting go. Do not bother your teenager with your problem of accepting untidiness. You have too many other important issues to negotiate, so do not waste your firepower. Tangential problems can arise out of this issue, though, and I suggest responding to them in the following way.

Leaves Clothes Outside the Bedroom

Do not pick them up and put them in the room or hang them in the closet. Have your teenager pick them up. If your teen refuses, get a large trash bag, hang it on the bedroom door, and throw clothes plus any other junk he or she leaves around the house into the bag.

Fails to Get Clothes to the Laundry Room

If clothes are not in the hamper or in the laundry room for weekly laundry, let your teen wash his or her own clothes or wear dirty ones. Remind your teen that he or she has a choice and that you accept whatever choice is made.

SIBLING FIGHTS

If your teenager is constantly arguing with siblings, do not get trapped into being a referee. As long as there is no physical touching, pushing, shoving, or hitting, tell them to take the arguments somewhere else where you do not have to hear the bickering. There is no cure for this one except to give yourself as much space from it as possible.

I realize, however, that some parents have trouble letting go of their wish to cure sibling rivalry. If you absolutely cannot stand it, separate the combatants from each other for half an hour. Sending them to their rooms is a good idea. Never ask who started it or let the kids tell you their side of the story. Unfortunately, there is little correlation between age and maturity in rivalry contests. Just be certain that no physical harm is taking place.

If your ADD teen is acting out anger or is physically aggressive with siblings, follow the steps outlined in Chapter 20.

CURFEW

As much as they may fight it, all teenagers need a curfew. I have talked to many teenagers who do not like their curfew, but prefer it to having no curfew at all. Younger teens, especially, tend to think that if their friends have lax curfews or no curfews at all, their friend's parents do not care about them. A curfew can give your teen a sense of safety and structure. Older teenagers need a curfew as well. Teens should not be left to come home whenever they please.

Setting a curfew should be done through a process of discussion. It is important to ask your youngster for ideas about curfew times and find out what your teen's friends' curfew times are. Be prepared in advance to have information about reasonable times so that you can set appropriate limits if your teenager asks for more time than you are comfortable allowing. You also need to show flexibility for special occasions and special circumstances. The rule is that you set the time if your teen cannot suggest a good curfew. Assuming the time you choose is fair, then the curfew is fixed and needs to be adhered to.

General rules of thumb are as follows.

1. Ages thirteen to fifteen stay home weeknights. Weekend curfew between 9:30 and 10:30 p.m., depending upon what children the same age are abiding by and your child's level of responsibility.
2. Ages sixteen and seventeen, 10:00 to 10:30 p.m. weeknights, provided homework is completed, 11:30 p.m. on weekends with a little variation if your teenager is responsible.
3. Ages eighteen and nineteen, more flexibility on weeknights if work is completed, weekends home by 1:00 a.m. If your teen is behaving responsibly, you can be flexible and let him or her set the times, within reason (before 1:30 or 2:00 a.m.).

It is also important to prepare for contingencies. You should have a discussion about the consequences of breaking curfew before that happens. The most typical consequences for breaking curfew are to make the curfew earlier for a short period of time or to ground the teen on a non-school night if the time violation is more serious.

A better method is to allow a ten- or fifteen-minute grace period after which the clock starts ticking. After fifteen minutes late your teen should be docked that number of minutes on the next free night. Unless he or she has a good excuse, any infractions greater than an hour should be paid back double time.

Do not punish violations excessively, and do not overreact emotionally if your child breaks curfew. Use your skills as a parent to treat this as a smaller problem and discuss it rationally with your teen.

HOMEWORK

Setting homework times depends upon the grades and attitudes of your teenager. If your teen is doing well in school and consistently gets homework completed, allow him or her the responsibility to decide when to study. If your teen has ADD, chances are that he or she will need some help structuring free time for study. My rule of thumb is work before play.

Most ADDers do best when they study after taking a brief break following school. The following guidelines should be helpful.

1. If your teen is taking medication for ADD, be sure that he or she is properly medicated when studying. Sometimes teens forget to take their noon dosage; other times they may need to take additional medication if they appear too distractible or hyperactive. Discuss this with your doctor.
2. Study time should be the same each day, if possible. If your teen says that no homework was assigned and his or her grades are poor, have your teen sit for one to one-and-one-half hours at study time reading school material or studying from magazines or newspapers.
3. Do not allow any phone interruptions or interruptions by siblings. If possible, allow your teen to study in his or her room or another designated quiet place.
4. Have your teen show you the finished assignment and review the work when it is completed.

5. Completing homework earns your teen the privilege of having free time. If it appears that homework is taking too long, check with the school to see what they consider to be the norm.
6. If your teen loses assignments, misunderstands, forgets to turn in material, claims no homework was assigned, plays while studying, or you suspect difficulties of this type, use the study checklists in Chapter 15, "Easing the Homework Struggle."

ADD teens frequently avoid or try to skip homework because it is boring and difficult for them. If your teenager is having trouble studying because he or she does not know how to organize work or is having trouble understanding assignments, it is important to help improve study habits. Most ADDers do not know how to study, organize, or prioritize their work. They lack the ability to distinguish between what is important and what is not important.

If you use the previous checklists, you will learn what types of problems your teenager is experiencing when sitting down to study. You may be able to help your teen learn to study; or you may want to seek assistance through the school; or you may want to engage a tutor to teach your teen how to learn. Discuss any of these issues with the school administration and see what resources are available to you. Review the information in Chapter 21, which discusses school problems and offers suggestions for helping your teenager through school.

TRUANCY

Truancy is a high-risk behavior. ADD teens who are truant are usually failing in school and having trouble at home. For immature teens, unstructured free time without supervision in school or at home usually leads to hanging out with peers who are bad influences. Drug use and trouble with the law may follow.

You need to work with the school, the truant officer, and your child to discover the problems. Frequently, the ADD teen who is truant is overwhelmed by schoolwork and is simply trying to escape. This problem can be dealt with in a variety of ways, depending on the circumstances. Traditional school may be more than your youngster can handle at this stage, in which case alternatives should be explored. Other times you may be able to work with your teen's school and have lessons modified, or an IEP plan can be developed (discussed in Chapter 14). Sometimes an alternative high school or home study program can be more appropriate.

Focus on solving the underlying causes of your teen's truancy. If you need professional help, consider counseling or other services available in your community. Most counties have low-cost agencies that provide counseling to families whose budgets are stretched.

While you are dealing with this problem, you should establish stern consequences for truant behavior. Grounding on weekends, removal of car privileges, and discontinuance of allowance are privileges that can be taken away until they are earned back by attending school again. In the meantime, you can work on the underlying issues creating the truancy.

Be alert to too many headaches, pains, and illnesses that your child uses as an excuse to stay home from school. A teen can attend school even if he or she has a cold or is feeling out of sorts.

Many ADD children show symptoms of depression or anxiety as they move into their teen years. If you notice sleep disturbances, dark moods, lack of energy, and similar symptoms, your teen may be experiencing emotional or psychological difficulties that require professional treatment.

Truancy is a serious problem that must be dealt with as soon as it is discovered. Your teenager will make excuses or attempt to manipulate you with tales of social alienation at school or mistreatment by a teacher. Stick to your guns; these things happen but they do not justify truancy. A serious discussion and the removal of privileges should be your first step as you focus on problem solving.

OUT OF CONTROL

There are two types of problems you might experience with your teenager if he or she is really out of control. One involves breaking the law. The second is running away. Both problems can be serious.

Breaking the Law

Some ADD teens seem to have a propensity for tangling with the law. Infractions can vary from relatively minor incidents to very serious ones. You must be on your toes to manage the serious incidents and to make sure that the less serious encounters are handled well.

One example of a minor incident is breaking curfew and being taken home by the police. Or the police may bring your teen home if he or she appears to be drunk in a public place. Just recently a teenager I counsel told me that he and a friend were making bets that the other one would not "moon" cars. My young patient decided to take up the bet. After mooning cars for about ten minutes, a police officer drove by and caught sight of the teen's derriere. The young man was promptly taken home to his mother. His embarrassment was punishment enough.

Unfortunately, some youngsters get picked up for more serious charges. Within the past two years, two of my patients were picked up for stealing and breaking and entering. In the first case, the youngster had already passed through the legal system and was referred to me by his probation officer. By the time he reached me, after spending time incarcerated, he had already decided to stop seeing his old friends and was on his way to becoming more responsible.

In another case, a youngster I worked with had a very difficult time with his mother, who would fly off the handle for minor infractions. Once, she grounded her son for a period of months for a small incident. He could not stand the confinement with no end in sight and, acting out his rage, broke into a store and stole some items. The police immediately apprehended him and his friends. In court, they made amends and returned or made good on all broken property. None of the youngsters received any jail time. My patient was told that when he was eighteen years of age his record would be expunged.

A few years elapsed and my young friend became very interested in the Navy Seals. He spent several weeks at their recruitment center and was eager to enter the military. He was ready to sign a contract to enter the Navy when he graduated from high school, but the Navy turned him down because of his felony arrest a few years earlier. He was completely heartbroken. It was a shame for this eager young man and for the Navy because he was a very intelligent and hard-working youngster.

ADD teens are particularly impulsive and sometimes act out in very immature ways, as did the young man above. Unfortunately, the effects of such reactions can be quite costly in the long run.

In many cases, breaking the law can result in your teen going to jail or juvenile hall. I have worked with a number of youngsters picked up while using or dealing marijuana. Many of them were sentenced to a probationary period and drug counseling; however, some do get sentenced to jail and a few unfortunates end up with a felony record as an adult.

Recently, I worked with a young man who was caught with a small amount of marijuana and some speed in his pocket. He came for therapy and I found that he was struggling with depression and a very serious ADD problem. He responded rapidly to medication and counseling. Both his psychiatrist and I wrote letters to persuade the judge to give this young man a second chance and the court refused. He was sentenced to jail for six months.

The best method for avoiding confrontation with the law is prevention. In the previously cited case histories, the children were well into their teens before professional intervention was sought. Children display numerous signs of having trouble over the years, long before they start breaking the law. Good communication between parents and children is essential to avoid the escalation of acting-out behavior. As a child begins to show signs of oppositional defiant disorder or conduct disorder, discussed in Chapter 20, professional help should be sought.

Running Away

When teens cannot get along with their families they are at high risk of running away, particularly if they have a conduct disorder with ADD. Most runaways are already using drugs, which compounds the seriousness of the dangers they might encounter.

More than one million teens run away each year. Teens who run do so because they have poor self-esteem, and because they believe the family does not care about them. Fewer run away because of physical or sexual abuse. ADD teens are at high risk because of their impulsiveness and because they feel desperate to find a quick solution to the ongoing problems which overwhelm them.

In a sense, when a child runs away it indicates that the family was not able to cope with the demands placed on them. The following guidelines may help parents deal with this problem.

1. When your youngster returns home after running away, insist that he or she attend family therapy sessions with you to work out agreements that all of you can live with. Remember that the best prognosis for working through this problem requires parents and children be prepared to make changes.
2. Sometimes you can arrange for your child to stay with a friend, relative, or neighbor for a cooling-off period. I had a youngster do very well when he moved from Napa to Santa Clara to live

with his uncle. He distanced himself from his old friends and found that he was able to start a new school and social life without his old connections pulling him down.

3. If you have trouble being firm with your ADD teen or setting limits and enforcing them, you may find help through a support group. Tough Love is a group of adults who are challenged by their children and meet to support one another. They find it helpful to gain support and share experiences working with their challenges. It is not unusual for a member to volunteer to take another member's child for awhile.

4. The youngster I mentioned previously who was not able to get into the Navy made an arrangement to live with friends for a period of time. I find that troubled teens tend to be more respectful and careful with other adults, such as a friend's parents, than they are with their own parents.

5. Parents may find a boarding school or military school to be a helpful alternative for their child. There are also schools that specialize in the education and treatment of ADD children.

When dealing with these issues, parents need to seek guidance from a professional, whether or not the child participates in the sessions. Parents need to determine limits to set and communicate this information to their teen so that the child knows what to expect when returning home. The professional can help the parents stick to their guns.

In the first chapter of this book, I discussed my daughter, Manuela. She ran away fifteen or twenty times until we followed the advice of our therapists. It was a very difficult time for us but we made it and, in time, Manuela came back to live with us. When she came back, she stuck to her agreements to attend school which somewhat surprised me.

More serious problems such as truancy, running away, or trouble with the law should be managed like any other problems your ADD teen creates. Your focus should be on resolving the problem and, as much as you are able, on setting your emotions aside. To do this you need to have as much information as possible about the incident, follow the suggestions on communication outlined in Chapter 19, and seek professional help.

When working with your ADD teenager there may be times when you can benefit from professional assistance. This assistance need not be expensive. Most cities have excellent family service agencies, low-cost community drug counseling, CHAAD groups, as well as professionals who specialize in the treatment of ADD problems. It is a good idea to obtain information about the resources available in your area so that you can call on them should the need arise.

LEARNING TO STEP BACK

As much as possible, step back from daily problems. The less ego involvement you have with getting your teen to comply with your wishes, the easier it will be. To help you with this, try to imagine that you have been given stewardship of your youngster for a short period of time. During this time you are called upon for counsel and guidance so that one day your child will be able to take responsibility for his or her own life and build both self-confidence and self-esteem. You are doing this not just by demanding compliance with your wishes but by having your child develop important personal skills.

As you learn to accept your ADD teen as a person with special challenges that sometimes bring out the worst in him or her, the easier it will be for you to place your teen's actions in perspective. No matter how it might appear at times, your ADD teenager is sensitive. When you are able to hold the perspective described here and communicate it to your teen, he or she will know that you care about your child. But do not be too hard on yourself in the process. It is impossible to maintain acceptance and love for anyone all of the time, let alone a difficult teenager. The more that you can learn to step back and let go of your attachment to a particular standard of behavior, the better off you will be. Your acceptance tells your teen that there is room, with your guidance, to build skills and develop self-esteem so that one day he or she might win this perplexing struggle.

Index

Page numbers followed by the letter "f" indicate figures.

Order Your Own Copy of
This Important Book for Your Personal Library!

WILD CHILD
How You Can Help Your Child with Attention Deficit Disorder (ADD) and Other Behavioral Disorders

_____in hardbound at $59.95 (ISBN: 0-7890-1101-8)
_____in softbound at $18.95 (ISBN: 0-7890-1102-6)

COST OF BOOKS_____

OUTSIDE USA/CANADA/
MEXICO: ADD 20%____

POSTAGE & HANDLING_____
(US: $4.00 for first book & $1.50
for each additional book)
Outside US: $5.00 for first book
& $2.00 for each additional book)

SUBTOTAL_____

in Canada: add 7% GST____

STATE TAX____
(NY, OH & MIN residents, please
add appropriate local sales tax)

FINAL TOTAL____
(If paying in Canadian funds,
convert using the current
exchange rate, UNESCO
coupons welcome.)

❑ **BILL ME LATER:** ($5 service charge will be added)
(Bill-me option is good on US/Canada/Mexico orders only;
not good to jobbers, wholesalers, or subscription agencies.)

❑ Check here if billing address is different from
shipping address and attach purchase order and
billing address information.

Signature_____

❑ **PAYMENT ENCLOSED: $**_____

❑ **PLEASE CHARGE TO MY CREDIT CARD.**

❑ Visa ❑ MasterCard ❑ AmEx ❑ Discover
❑ Diner's Club ❑ Eurocard ❑ JCB

Account # _____

Exp. Date_____

Signature_____

Prices in US dollars and subject to change without notice.

NAME_____

INSTITUTION_____

ADDRESS_____

CITY_____

STATE/ZIP_____

COUNTRY_____ COUNTY (NY residents only)_____

TEL_____ FAX_____

E-MAIL_____

May we use your e-mail address for confirmations and other types of information? ❑ Yes ❑ No
We appreciate receiving your e-mail address and fax number. Haworth would like to e-mail or fax special
discount offers to you, as a preferred customer. **We will never share, rent, or exchange your e-mail address
or fax number.** We regard such actions as an invasion of your privacy.

Order From Your Local Bookstore or Directly From
The Haworth Press, Inc.
10 Alice Street, Binghamton, New York 13904-1580 • USA
TELEPHONE: 1-800-HAWORTH (1-800-429-6784) / Outside US/Canada: (607) 722-5857
FAX: 1-800-895-0582 / Outside US/Canada: (607) 722-6362
E-mail: getinfo@haworthpressinc.com
PLEASE PHOTOCOPY THIS FORM FOR YOUR PERSONAL USE.
www.HaworthPress.com